ESSENTIALS

COMMUNICATION SKILLS

For Nursing and Healthcare Students

ESSENTIALS

COMMUNICATION SKILLS

For Nursing and Healthcare Students

Edited by
KAY NORMAN

Lantern

ISBN: 9781908625779

Lantern Publishing Ltd, The Old Hayloft, Vantage Business Park, Bloxham Rd, Banbury, OX16 9UX, UK
www.lanternpublishing.com

www.cla.co.uk

British Library Cataloguing in Publication Data
A catalogue record for this book is available from the British Library

The authors and publisher have made every attempt to ensure the content of this book is up to date
and accurate. However, healthcare knowledge and information is changing all the time so the reader
is advised to double-check any information in this text on drug usage, treatment procedures, the use
of equipment, etc. to confirm that it complies with the latest safety recommendations, standards of
practice and legislation, as well as local Trust policies and procedures. Students are advised to check
with their tutor and/or practice supervisor before carrying out any of the procedures in this textbook.

Cover design by Andrew Magee Design Ltd
Cover image reproduced under licence from stock.adobe.com
Typeset by Medlar Publishing Solutions Pvt Ltd, India
Printed in the UK
Last digit is the print number: 10 9 8 7 6 5

Contents

About the authors

Dr Kay Norman is Head of Department for Practice Learning and Partnerships at The University of Worcester.

Kay has held senior clinical, academic and management posts in nursing within a variety of healthcare organisations and universities. As a Registered Nurse and Specialist Practitioner, her clinical background focused on primary care and community nursing. Her current role involves working with practice partners, students and academic staff to deliver innovative learning experiences for pre-registration nursing students. Kay's research interests include the image of nursing, coaching and supervision in practice, and nursing leadership/teamwork. She has published in peer-reviewed journals, written various book chapters and edited a professional portfolio textbook, and presented her research at international conferences.

Louise Carter is a Senior Lecturer in adult nursing at the University of Worcester. Before moving into education, she held clinical posts in medical, surgical and community nursing, enjoying over 20 years of caring for patients. With a passion for teaching and supporting others, Louise also worked as a Practice Facilitator, advocating for both students and mentors. She has a particular interest in clinical skills and simulation teaching, and the development of innovative ways to deliver practice learning. Louise combines her role in the classroom with that of Induction Tutor for the BSc (Hons) Nursing programme.

Alison Lewis currently works as a Senior Lecturer at the University of Worcester. Alison has worked extensively within the public health nursing field for over 20 years, where she specialised in promoting access to primary care for homeless and non-English-speaking families. Prior to joining the University of Worcester, Alison worked within the Family Nurse Partnership programme supporting teenage parents and their babies. She has recently published research investigating how public health nurses support young people who are experiencing negative aspects of 'sexting', and holds the Queen's Nurse title, which recognises community nurses who have shown a high level of commitment to patient care and nursing practice.

Val Nixon is Head of Department for Adult Nursing at the University of Worcester. Val qualified as a Registered Nurse in 1993 and gained extensive clinical experience in emergency nursing, before embarking on her career in higher education in 2004. Within varying academic posts in higher education, Val has worked across both pre- and post-registration nursing and paramedic programmes and more recently, the nursing associate programme. Val has a special interest in patient safety, which is the theme of her PhD study. Val has previous experience of publishing, through a number of publications in peer-reviewed journals, book editor and author of book chapters.

Dr Pádraig Ó Lúanaigh is Director of Nursing at Mayo University Hospital, Ireland. With over 30 years' experience of working within health and higher education, Pádraig has a broad and integrated range of experiences gained from working in organisations in several countries. With professional registrations as a nurse, midwife and health visitor and experience of working in primary and secondary care, he has a credible knowledge of leading provider and operational aspects of healthcare services. Pádraig has held teaching and leadership roles in education, complemented by strategic leadership and health policy experience in central government and strategic health organisations. Pádraig continues to publish and research a range of topics reflecting his professional background and has edited two international best-selling academic textbooks.

Erica Pavord is a Lecturer in Child and Adolescent Mental Health at the University of Worcester and works as a systemic counsellor with families in Monmouthshire. She has a special interest in communication methods and teaches a range of therapeutic communication and counselling skills. She has co-written two books: *An Introduction to Child and Adolescent Mental Health* by Burton, Pavord and Williams and *Communication and Interpersonal Skills* by Pavord and Donnelly. Her research interests include understanding attachment narratives and narrative inquiry methods.

Dr Naomi Anna Watson is a Lecturer in the Faculty of Wellbeing, Education and Language Studies at The Open University. Naomi has practised as a Registered Nurse, Senior Midwife and Specialist Practitioner Health Visiting. She is also a practice educator and Registered Nurse tutor. She has researched, written and published in primary care nursing, public health, diversity, ethnicity, cultural competence, service user involvement, nursing education and black women's health and wellbeing. Naomi is also an Associate Editor of the *Journal of Ethnicity and Health* and has a keen interest in natural health and healing in diverse communities. Naomi's research interests include cultural competence in healthcare and education, diversity and ethnicity, and experiences of black, British African Caribbean people about nursing careers.

Introduction

This book is designed primarily for student nurses who care for adult patients, and will help you to appreciate the many facets of communication in your role. You are obviously interested in progressing your understanding of communication skills by reading this book, so hopefully the various chapters will encourage you to question your own communication practices, as well as those of others, to learn and improve together. This reading will require you to take time to think critically, challenge you to question your own viewpoints and approaches, and to reflect on past and current situations where communication encounters may have gone well or not so well. Reflective activities are included in each chapter to help you apply your learning to practice situations.

Ultimately you are responsible for upholding the professional standards within the Nursing and Midwifery Council (NMC) *Code*. The four areas – prioritise people, practise effectively, preserve safety, and promote professionalism and trust – all have communication at the heart of their section statements, and are evidenced throughout all chapters of this book. As a student nurse in 1986 I remember the first quote I had to memorise: "Communication is the essence of nursing", which still holds true today. Communication as a concept is fundamental to the nursing profession and must be nurtured and practised.

Communication methods are many and varied, with additional texts available on specific areas, such as social media and technological aspects. This book will focus on the themes included in the NMC (2018) *Standards for Pre-registration Nursing* (Annexe A). Each chapter will provide you with some detailed information and activities to develop your learning and understanding. Key learning points and further reading resources are highlighted at the end of each chapter. Many chapters also include websites and video clips that support the reading material. Case studies draw together the main concepts and themes discussed in each chapter, providing reflective questions to evaluate your learning.

All chapter authors have a wealth of practice and educational experience and are passionate about sharing their communication expertise with you. We do hope you enjoy your reading and learning journey.

Kay Norman, Editor

Chapter 1

Communication as a concept

Kay Norman and Erica Pavord

LEARNING OUTCOMES

By the end of this chapter you should be able to:

1.1 Have an understanding of the various communication modes and channels used in society

1.2 Have an awareness of relevant communication frameworks and how these reflect human interaction

1.3 Appreciate the importance of self-awareness and reflection in the communication process

1.4 Apply your learning to nursing practice.

1.1 Introduction

Communication can be seen as fundamental to all nursing care and activity. As the world of healthcare continually changes, it is more important than ever for nurses to adapt and perfect their communication skills to provide effective, ethical care. The NMC *Code* (Nursing and Midwifery Council, 2018a) refers to communication in many of its professional standards. Alongside this, the NMC standards of proficiency for registered nurses (Nursing and Midwifery Council, 2018b) outline the communication and relationship skills that a newly registered nurse must be able to demonstrate in order to meet the required proficiency outcomes. Therefore, defining and understanding the concept of communication is the first stage in scaffolding your learning around this central aspect of person-centred care. This chapter does not aim to review all the available communication theories from a range of disciplines, but it will explore some of the relevant frameworks that can help us as nurses understand how we interact with each other and with patients/carers. It will also discuss the importance of self-awareness and reflection in the communication process.

1.2 Defining communication

As a profession whose main activity involves interacting with others in some way, whether that be with patients, carers, the general public, team members, or each other, nursing should be seen as role modelling a gold standard of communication. Communication in building a therapeutic relationship, as part of assessment, accurate recording, providing clear information/instructions, engaging in difficult conversations, accommodating communication impairments, and ultimately demonstrating compassion, are just a few areas of nursing care where this concept is seen. However, communication is a complex concept with no single definition and, depending on the context, can mean different things to different people.

Within healthcare, good communication is constantly referred to as underpinning all episodes of care. The NHS Constitution (Department of Health and Social Care, 2015) consists of key principles to guide the NHS, which are based on core NHS values, all of which require some level of effective communication to be achieved. The subsequent 6Cs (described by the Clinical Leaders Network: www.cln.nhs. uk/6csforeveryone/what-are-the-6cs?.html) are the value base for *Leading Change, Adding Value: a framework for nursing, midwifery and care staff*, which also relies on effective communication for all values to be realised (NHS England, 2016). The framework identifies ten commitments to demonstrate impact and success, reduce variation in care, and to ensure these values are embedded in care culture. The 6Cs are:

■ **Care**

Care is our core business and that of our organisations and the care we deliver helps the individual person and improves the health of the whole community. Caring defines us and our work. People receiving care expect it to be right for them consistently throughout every stage of their life.

■ **Compassion**

Compassion is how care is given through relationships based on empathy, respect and dignity; it can also be described as intelligent kindness and is central to how people perceive their care.

■ **Competence**

Competence means all those in caring roles must have the ability to understand an individual's health and social needs and the expertise, clinical and technical knowledge to deliver effective care and treatments based on research and evidence.

■ **Communication**

Communication is central to successful caring relationships and to effective teamworking. Listening is as important as what we say and do and essential for 'no decision about me without me'. Communication is the key to a good workplace with benefits for staff and patients alike.

■ Courage

Courage enables us to do the right thing for the people we care for, to speak up when we have concerns and to have the personal strength and vision to innovate and to embrace new ways of working.

■ Commitment

A commitment to our patients and populations is a cornerstone of what we do. We need to build on our commitment to improve the care and experience of our patients to take action to make this vision and strategy a reality for all and meet the health and social care challenges ahead.

It has been established that effective communication is fundamental in all nursing activity, yet we are constantly reminded that communication goes wrong in many instances. Media reports often highlight the lack of communication between healthcare staff and patients which leads to errors, with communication problems remaining one of the most common causes of complaint in UK health services. Reader *et al.* (2014) reported that complaints about problematic communication and poor staff–patient relationships were almost as frequent as those concerning quality of care.

So, what do we mean by 'communication'? Begin by thinking about your own understanding of this term.

ACTIVITY 1.1

What does communication mean to you? Make a list of words that come to mind when you think of communication. It might help to reflect on all communication episodes you have encountered today or within the last week. Try to think about the different types and methods of communication you have experienced in a variety of contexts. From this, write a working definition that is meaningful to you.

We all have our own personal understanding of what communication is but it will probably involve some reference to the definition from the Collins English Dictionary: "The imparting or exchange of information, ideas or feelings."

You may have considered communication as a two-way process or as involving others in some way. The process of communication exists in all humans, whether it is voluntary or involuntary. Gault *et al.* (2017, p. 16) suggest that "Communication is a complex interaction…cyclical in nature, allowing a message to be sent and received, following which there will be either confirmation of receipt of the information or interpretation of the interaction as successful or otherwise."

Communication can be both verbal and non-verbal, involving a wide range of methods and channels. Review the word cloud in *Figure 1.1* for similarities to your own list of communication words from *Activity 1.1*. This is not an exhaustive list, but we can clearly appreciate there are multiple ways of communicating.

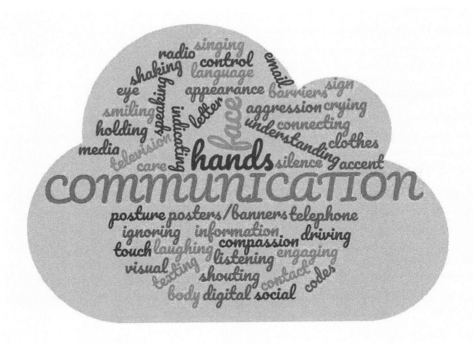

Figure 1.1 *Word cloud based around 'communication' methods and channels.*

1.3 Communication frameworks

We use different modes of communication depending on the context. For example, a chat with friends via social media will be different to a professional conversation as part of an interview, or supporting a patient and their relatives in the final stages of their illness. It is important to be aware of the type of approach you choose in order to be effective in communicating the intended message. Having some understanding of communications theory and frameworks can help determine the most effective strategy to use.

There are four main frameworks for theories of communication. These are:

- **Mechanistic** – this framework was originally used by people working on radio and telephone communications and incorporates a transmission model of communication.
- **Psychological** – this framework concentrates far more on how we feel during a communication and our emotional responses.
- **Social constructionist** – this framework is concerned with how we all construct different realities from the same experiences.
- **Systemic** – this framework concentrates on the way that communication is part of a whole system and how, within that system, each part of the communication is repeatedly re-examined and reworked.

We will look at two models of communication within these frameworks. The first is a transmission model. This type of model is included in the mechanistic framework and is said to be linear in its process. It is a simple straightforward model that is easy to understand and can be very useful in helping analyse communication processes between people and organisations.

The second model to be considered is a transactional model, which combines principles from the psychological, social constructionist and systemic frameworks. The transactional model is more complicated than the mechanistic one and further explores the experience of shared meanings in our communications with others.

1.4 The transmission model

One of the earliest, most basic and well-known communication models is that of Shannon and Weaver (1949). Their model is sometimes referred to as the 'mother of communication models' and it provides a good starting point for anyone studying communication theory.

As you can see in *Figure 1.2*, the arrows that show transmission from the information source to the destination point in only one direction, reflecting the belief that messages flow in only one direction at any given time. It is therefore a linear process.

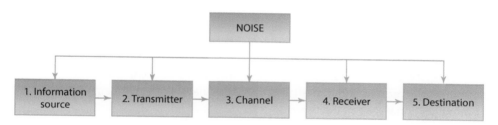

Figure 1.2 *The Shannon and Weaver transmission model.*

The Shannon and Weaver model consists of five parts and what they term 'noise'. In a face-to-face communication:
1. The information would be the idea that you had in your head.
2. The transmitter would be you sending the message.
3. The channel would be your voice as you speak the idea.
4. The receiver would be the ear of the person to whom you are talking.
5. The destination would be the intended person's head.

Noise, as you can see, can occur at any point within that communication process, and can prevent the original thought or idea reaching its destination intact and as intended.

Noise can be anything. Noise might be:
- Physical, i.e. what we commonly call noise – a loud sound (physical noise).
- Psychological, i.e. an emotion such as anxiety or a strongly-held point of view or a cultural barrier (psychological noise).

- Semantic, i.e. a language or representation problem (semantic noise).
- Physiological, i.e. deafness, blindness or pain (physiological noise).

Noise can interrupt the communication at any stage.

If your message is not getting across, this simple model gives you the opportunity to explore some of the reasons why. Once the 'noise' is identified you can then try to eliminate or at least modify the 'noise' or message in some way. The possibilities are all subject to the nature of the 'noise' and may require you to do some strategic thinking and extra planning to ensure your message gets across. Can you think of any recent examples of 'noise' interfering with a message you wanted to convey? Never believe that people have heard exactly what you meant to say without first checking their understanding and making sure the message reached its destination intact and as you intended it. Using such a simple strategy will help avoid all sorts of complications later on.

1.5 The transactional model

Another model of communication is a transactional model developed by Julia Wood (2004). She defines communication as: "…a systemic process in which individuals interact with and through symbols to create and interpret meanings" (Wood, 2004), and offers the following diagram (*Figure 1.3*) to illustrate communications taking place between two people.

In this model you can see that communicator A transmits a message to communicator B, who receives the message, decodes the message, has a reaction to the message and then responds to communicator A. Notice that the 'noise' surrounds the process and that 'shared messages' have a direct impact on the communication between the two.

This is a far more complex model of communication than that of Shannon and Weaver, which was linear in its process. In this model messages are being sent backwards and forwards all the time, not just in one direction but simultaneously. The transactional model focuses on how we interpret meaning and how meanings are shared within our communication with other people.

When communication goes wrong it is often the result of meaning being misinterpreted. Meaning in communication is said to be negotiated between the people concerned. For example, if you use a word in one context with friends it will be interpreted in a particular way by that social group but, use the same word or communication with your teachers or parents, and the meaning is not shared on the same level. For example, the words 'sick', 'whatever' and 'random' come to mind, as we know older people's interpretations of these words are completely different from those of younger people. There are, no doubt, lots of other examples you can think of. Our language is constantly developing and has to accommodate new ways of living, new technologies and new ways of expressing feelings and thoughts. Social groups use a common language to communicate on a psychological and sociological level that isn't always instantly apparent to people on the outside of that group.

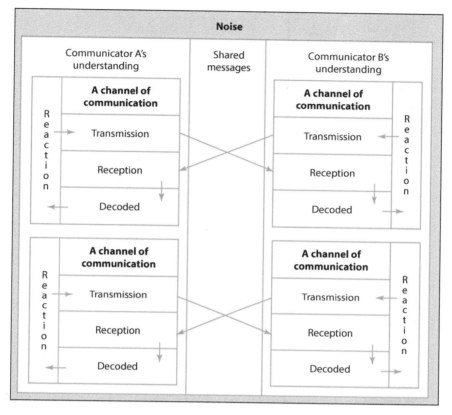

Figure 1.3 *The transactional model.*

The language we use, our non-verbal behaviours and the symbols we include in our communications all play a powerful role in establishing and sharing meaning. It is important to remember that understanding something is a subjective experience.

We construct meaning in social contexts and share a mutual awareness and often a mutual language that is culturally bound and age-related.

The transactional model is a more accurate model of what really happens in face-to-face communication than the Shannon and Weaver model. The transactional model takes into consideration all the aspects of communication that we looked at earlier in this chapter. It is also a better basis for any new communication system you might consider creating to help the people you work with. What is it in the transactional model that makes it so much better at explaining what real-life communication is like? The answer lies in the channels of communication.

1.6 **Channels of communication**

Multiple channels are being used in the transactional model. For example:
- facial expressions
- body angle

- posture
- presentation
- tone of voice
- words
- word images
- role portrayal.

If you refer back to *Figure 1.3* you will see that not only are multiple channels being used, but the arrows point both ways instead of in just one direction. The person sending the message is at the same time receiving a message through the same channels. As each person receives a message, they are simultaneously decoding it. They are using all their previous experiences and memories to sift through what they are receiving in order to give meaning to it. At the same time, they are creating and sending their own message and there is still all that 'noise' going on around the communications being sent, received and decoded.

There are a number of channels that we use to communicate with others. These channels or methods tend to correspond to particular senses such as sight and hearing and, for each channel that we use, there is a method or way that facilitates its use best. We all communicate in many different forms, and the methods available for us to communicate are always increasing as information and communication technology develops, providing us with the opportunity to use multiple channels of communication to get our messages across. All the channels or methods have different advantages and disadvantages. When choosing a way to communicate, some of the aspects that you need to take into consideration are:

- how much time is available
- how many people you are communicating with
- whether you want people to reply to you
- whether you want people to be able to ask you questions
- how much information you want to get from them
- how much information you want to give them
- how many senses (seeing, hearing, smelling) you need them to use for them to understand the information.

The way we choose to communicate with people depends on the channels of communication open to us. In a normal situation you do not notice yourself deciding on the considerations above when you communicate with someone. However, as someone working in a helping capacity in the health and social care fields, you do need to think more carefully about the best ways to communicate with someone else. You need to take into account their needs and not just yours, and balance those needs against the needs of the organisation you work within.

The message here is that once you start to unpick a communication and begin analysing the process, you can start to appreciate the depth of meaning that lies behind the words and actions that you engage in. Even if you try not to interact with others you are still communicating with them. By hiding in the back room/ office or just by simply staring out of the window you are communicating that you do not wish to interact with them. We communicate with all of our senses – our sight, hearing, smell and touch – in fact, we cannot *not* communicate, and in order to ensure that what we are communicating is appropriate, we need to be more consciously aware of the impact we have on others.

ACTIVITY 1.2

Choose three recent conversations – one with a friend or family member, one with a colleague or peer, and one with a manager or tutor. Use the frameworks above to analyse these communication encounters. What are the important points you have gained from this analysis and how will this inform your future communication practice?

1.7 Self-awareness in communication

From the models above it is recognised that we as individuals will communicate in many different ways. This will depend on our culture, language, experiences, values and beliefs. Communication is open to interpretation from the receiver, so the intended meaning can often become misconstrued. Awareness of the ways in which we communicate with others and the ways in which we respond to communication is important in considering our effectiveness in this process.

We may feel our message is clear but it is important to check for understanding. A rushed conversation with a patient asking how they are feeling, while looking at your watch, avoiding eye contact and with your arms folded, may not elicit an honest response. In addition, not offering important information in a team meeting due to lack of confidence or giving instructions to a colleague without explanation can result in serious unintended consequences. Issues resulting from poor communication have been consistently highlighted in health arenas, including the well-publicised Francis Report (2013) relating to the Mid-Staffordshire NHS Trust. The NHS continues to receive large numbers of complaints relating to communication errors and processes, which include both written and verbal communication (Parliamentary and Health Service Ombudsman, 2011). Therefore, developing self-awareness of your own communication style can help to identify where improvements can be made.

The NMC professional standards (Nursing and Midwifery Council, 2018b) include an annexe specifically relating to communication and interpersonal skills, where competence must be achieved to register as a nurse. The NMC *Code* (Nursing and

Midwifery Council, 2018a) also identifies communication within the standard below, although it is implicit throughout all standards:

PRACTISE EFFECTIVELY

7. Communicate clearly

7.1 Use terms that people in your care, colleagues and the public can understand

7.2 Take reasonable steps to meet people's language and communication needs, providing, wherever possible, assistance to those who need help to communicate their own or other people's needs

7.3 Use a range of verbal and non-verbal communication methods, and consider cultural sensitivities, to better understand and respond to people's personal and health needs

7.4 Check people's understanding from time to time to keep misunderstanding or mistakes to a minimum

7.5 Be able to communicate clearly and effectively in English

Various 'types' of communication are discussed in all chapters of this book, which will develop your understanding of how methods can be used in different situations. However, at this initial stage, it is useful to stop and consider your own communication style. It is often others' perspectives of how you communicate that can have the most impact in developing self-awareness. In this process, being aware of feelings, recognising characteristics that may influence behaviour, and a willingness to learn and change in order to improve the effectiveness of communication is essential. As mentioned earlier in this chapter, your fundamental values and belief systems can also impact on your attitudes and behaviour towards communication interactions, so need to be acknowledged and addressed accordingly.

ACTIVITY 1.3

Complete the SWEC (strengths, weaknesses, expectations, concerns) analysis in *Table 1.1* below, relating to your personal communication.

List ways in which you may be able to address the weaknesses and concerns and develop the expectations.

Following this, ask a variety of people (your supervisor, a colleague, fellow student, patients, friend, family member, etc.) to complete a similar SWEC for you, from their perspective, ensuring they are honest and constructive. If you include a patient, consent must be gained and this should be discussed with the appropriate placement manager.

Discuss these with your supervisor in order to produce a development plan.

Table 1.1 *SWEC analysis*

Strengths	Weaknesses
Expectations	Concerns

In order to develop self-awareness, it is important to receive honest and open feedback. This can sometimes be difficult to accept initially, especially if it conflicts with your own perceptions. Nevertheless, these views need to be considered carefully and discussed in depth with your supervisor to support your development going forward. This can also help to embed a culture of learning within the healthcare team, encouraging learning with and from each other, and accepting/ offering constructive feedback as a positive process. This is discussed further in *Chapter 7.*

It is also important to recognise external factors that can affect communication. If you are aware of these and how they might impact on communication processes, coping methods and strategies can be implemented. Some of the external factors that you might encounter are listed below. Can you think of any others?

- Lack of sleep/tiredness
- Hunger/thirst
- Emotional vulnerability
- Relationships
- Personal commitments
- Illness.

You may recognise the above areas as elements we would also consider in the assessment of a patient. In addition to recognising these factors as potentially impacting on your own communication, this can also relate to how others communicate with you (patients, colleagues, supervisors). In developing self-awareness, you can take steps to address these. For example, you may be quiet in a team meeting or appear distant when discussing a patient's needs with a colleague, or appear irritated with a year 1 student when they ask for help. In genuinely explaining the reasons you acted in this way and apologising, you can resolve a potential communication barrier with others and develop open, trusting relationships.

1.7.1 Emotional intelligence

Working in a healthcare environment can be rewarding but also challenging at times, and so it is important to recognise your limitations and ask for help when needed. Because the need to care is paramount, this can sometimes cloud judgement in respect of our own emotional and health needs. However, as self-awareness develops you will become better at identifying the way you are feeling and the potential impact it may have in your interactions with others. You may have heard of the term 'emotional intelligence', which has its roots in psychology and was further developed by Goleman (1996). This essentially describes a process concerned with interacting and empathising with others, where you are aware and in control of your emotions, managing them in a positive way. It consists of five key elements:

Self-awareness: Recognising and understanding your emotions and how these impact on self and others.

Self-regulation: Controlling emotions that could become destructive. Allowing space to consider negative emotions before acting upon them. Accepting alternative actions in the decision-making process, rather than acting impulsively in an emotionally charged situation. Acting with honesty and integrity.

Motivation: Recognising the positive elements in situations. Setting clear goals with optimism. Even if you feel negative thoughts arising at times, you can consciously reframe them in a more positive way.

Empathy: Recognising and acknowledging the situations of others, how and why they feel and behave the way they do. Helping others develop. In addition, considering how your own behaviours can influence and affect others.

Social skills: Developing interpersonal skills, building honest, transparent relationships, developing self-confidence, listening and engaging with others in a meaningful way, helping to work with others to develop solutions.

1.7.2 Mindfulness

Mindfulness is another tool that can be used to develop self-awareness. Studies have also suggested that practising mindfulness, including breathing techniques and meditation, can reduce stress and enhance a sense of wellbeing (Foureur et al., 2013; van der Riet et al., 2014). This practice originated in a spiritual context, but is now gaining momentum as a practice to adopt in many areas of life, including healthcare practice and specifically nursing (Escuriex and Labbé, 2012; Snowden et al., 2015). To practise mindfulness is to pay attention to the here and now – what we are feeling, thinking and doing, and how this is affecting us. Mindfulness practice is essentially focusing your attention on the present moment, accepting what it is without judgement.

We can all engage in this practice when we are relaxed or in comfortable surroundings. However, it is suggested that when we feel out of control, stressed, tired or preoccupied, this is more difficult to achieve. As healthcare professionals we are encouraged to reflect, although finding time for contemplation within a busy working environment is challenging and the desire to suppress feelings from patients and colleagues in order to 'get the job done' is commonplace (Sumner, 2010).

Much mindfulness literature suggests that core mindfulness concerns using the reasonable mind in combination with the emotional mind to harmonise a wise mind (*Figure 1.4*).

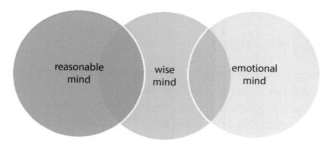

Figure 1.4 *Mindfulness states of mind.*

The **reasonable mind** refers to our rational self and is task-oriented. When in this state of mind, we are concerned with logic, facts and reason. Emotional detachment can be observed.

The **emotional mind** refers to how our emotions can dominate our thoughts. We can be ruled by our feelings and moods, with logic, facts and reason not seen as important. We can become over-emotional.

The **wise mind** refers to seeing the benefit and value of both the reasonable and emotional mind states. It is concerned with integrating both mindsets to achieve a balance. This suggests that in adopting this mind state, we will make better decisions.

There are many mindfulness texts and web material which discuss various approaches, including breathing techniques, taking technology time out, being grateful, appreciating the beauty around you. However, there are three main action areas to consider when implementing mindfulness:

Observe: becoming consciously aware and accepting of what is occurring without making a judgement as to whether it is good or bad.

Describe: naming all aspects of the experience that you are aware of, for example I'm experiencing anxiety, my face feels hot, my mouth is dry.

Participate: making a choice, taking action, acknowledging your feelings, taking the next step as consciously as you can. This is drawing on your own inner resources, rather than becoming a victim or resisting how you are feeling.

Practising the above areas has been linked to improving self-confidence in addition to self-awareness, although it does need commitment to embed this into everyday life (Walker and Mann, 2015). To find more information on mindfulness and six simple exercises to try, access Pocket Mindfulness at: www.pocketmindfulness.com/6-mindfulness-exercises-you-can-try-today/

Be kind to yourself and accept who you are in your journey to access your full potential. It is important to realise you are not superhuman and with help and support, you can learn to analyse and adapt to situations as they occur. As you gain self-insight by observing your own thinking and actions, rather than judging, your communication with both patients and colleagues will improve. In professional practice you will subsequently become more accepting of others and adopt non-judgemental care approaches.

1.8 Reflective practice

In order to learn from experiences to make improvements, we must consider the relevant situation or scenario in sufficient depth to make sense of the issues involved. In essence this is reflective practice. Many reflective frameworks and models are used in healthcare to help organise and structure our thoughts and feelings. However, in nursing education, it has been suggested that reflective practice can be difficult to 'teach' and the idea of academic reflections as forms of assessment can be detrimental to embedding a culture of reflection in practice. Nevertheless, it is important that reflective practice is seen positively in nursing and is seen as an 'inquiry' process to consider alternatives and propose change. The NMC has also included a requirement for reflection within their revalidation process, so all nurses must embrace this concept to examine their learning.

Schön (1983) is seen as the most influential writer on reflection. He proposed two elements of reflective practice. 'Reflection on action' refers to considering an event at a later point. This may be through personal contemplation, writing notes of feelings, what went well, what could be improved. 'Reflection in action' refers to responding to an event as it happens, drawing on previous experience or knowledge to influence practice. Reflection in action can then be considered as reflection on action at a later stage.

It is not the aim of this chapter to discuss all models and processes of reflective practice as there are many texts available which specifically focus on this subject area. However, it is necessary to discuss some of the models available here and how these can be used as part of the communication process. Boud (2010) suggests that reflection is fundamental to the nursing profession as there is a particular emphasis on the interaction between professional and patient. Therefore, it is the responsibility of all individuals, teams and the organisation to reflect and learn from practice in order to develop and improve patient care and services.

We all reflect on experiences in our lives informally, but to critically reflect in our professional roles requires linking theory to practice and involves structured, conscious thought (Oelofsen, 2012). This allows for a more evidenced approach to improving practice and in turn, develops self-awareness and encourages positive change (Savage, 2013). The most commonly used reflective model in nursing is the Gibbs (1988) reflective cycle, as shown in *Figure 1.5*.

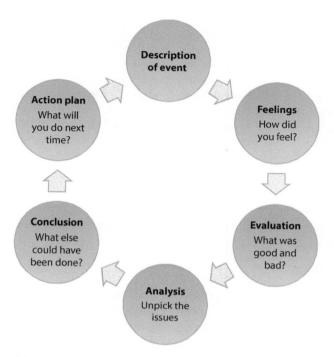

Figure 1.5 *The Gibbs reflective cycle.*

The Gibbs model prompts a more analytical approach to reflecting on an event or situation. Although it initially asks for a description of the event, critical thinking aspects of evaluation and analysis are used to unpick the issues involved to develop actions for future improvement. This model is often used as a chosen framework for academic writing as part of reflective assessments.

Borton's development framework (Borton, 1970) is a simple guide to reflective activities but still requires critical thinking to make sense of the specific situation. It consists of three questions:

What   have I learned?

did I hope to learn?

surprised me?

So what   is the importance of this learning?

more do I need to know about this?

have I learnt about this?

Now what   can I do?

do I need to do?

might I do to improve or enhance the care I deliver to patients?

might be the consequences of this action?

ACTIVITY 1.4

Using both reflective frameworks above, reflect on a recent communication encounter with a patient that didn't go as well as you thought. Identify the particular issues involved. Consider all elements of the frameworks to develop a plan for future improvement. Discuss this with your supervisor to share your learning and gain their thoughts and perspectives. How did both models help you look at the issues in sufficient depth to learn and improve from this experience?

You can practise using various models of reflection in order to choose the most suitable for you. Whichever model you decide to use, the focus should be about effecting and enabling change, whether that be a personal change in you, such as adopting a different communication strategy, or influencing change of a service or team through sharing your reflections and proposed actions.

1.8.1 Think aloud

Reflective activities can be just as powerful, if not more so, if done as part of a group or team. By reflecting together on specific case studies, incidents and scenarios in practice, groups can build an open, transparent culture that acknowledges everyone's interpretation and perspective. Think aloud (TA) is also a strategy that can be used within group reflections and has been successfully used as part of clinical skills and simulation activities, where nursing students are encouraged to verbalise their thoughts whilst completing the simulation task and also retrospectively. This has encouraged confidence in clinical reasoning and improved articulation when discussing care (Burbach *et al.*, 2015). Tanner (2006) has suggested that retrospective TA is also critical in sound judgement formation to clarify thinking and analyse communication patterns.

TA as a learning strategy focuses on encouraging you to have a mental representation of a scenario to clarify clinical thinking. When used regularly, this strategy helps to build mental pictures of situations and how to consider and progress to a possible solution, which can be subsequently drawn upon in the future. When we think of any word, for example car, our brains immediately conjure up meaning, images and feelings associated with that word. This is ultimately how humans learn and react, and how perceptions are formed and become structures of our reality. In a clinical situation, this verbal TA strategy can help to improve and understand the mental processes we are using to formulate a decision in a logical way. It has also been suggested that this strategy contributes to the development of memory through verbalisation when reflecting after an event.

CASE STUDY

You are due to work with the community nursing team as part of your year 1 placement experience. You are enthusiastic but a little apprehensive about delivering nursing care in people's homes.

You have tried to contact the team and have left several messages to arrange a pre-placement visit but have received no response. On the first day you arrive at the team base at 09.00 and your identified supervisor has left for visits. You are informed the team start at 08.30.

What actions could you have taken to prevent this? What methods of communication might now be suitable in this situation?

You decide to make the most of the time at the base to explore the learning environment and read around the types of nursing care delivered in the community nursing team. The administrator gives you relevant literature and an access code for the intranet. Your supervisor returns at lunchtime and discusses your identified needs and possible learning experiences to achieve your proficiencies. You have many questions from your reading and also require some clarification on Trust policies, so begin to read the list you have made. Your supervisor folds her arms and seems a little irritated and explains that afternoon visits must take priority now.

What would you consider as appropriate next steps in this situation? Explore possible aspects of your own and your supervisor's communication methods.

Your supervisor drives to the next visit and discusses information about the next patient you will see, who has limited mobility and needs a wound dressing change. On arrival, the patient's daughter offers you a drink and informs your supervisor that her mother's wound is now becoming very painful. As your supervisor continues to assess and dress the wound, the daughter begins to cry.

What would you do in this situation? What communication methods would you draw on?

On the way back to base, your supervisor discusses the types of treatment used, side effects and pain relief medication. However, you can only think about how upset the daughter seemed and whether you had managed to help in any way. The following day your supervisor asks you to recap the information she had given you the day before regarding treatments and medications but you have forgotten.

What would be your action points?

What would you do if a similar episode were to occur in the future?

Summary

Effective communication can be seen as the essence of nursing and underpins all that we do as nurses, relating to knowledge acquisition, skills and behaviours. Understanding models and theories of communication helps to develop a critical viewpoint of our own and others' communication in order to improve. Advancing self-awareness through techniques such as mindfulness and reflection can help you take ownership of communication encounters and generate solutions for future episodes of care.

KEY LEARNING POINTS

Three key points to take away from *Chapter 1*:

- ☑ Communication is not only concerned with verbal interaction. It covers a multitude of mediums, incorporating verbal and non-verbal mechanisms.
- ☑ A variety of communication methods can be drawn upon for successful interaction, depending on the situation. Consider combinations of these methods in episodes of care.
- ☑ Development of self-awareness and reflection skills can help to enhance and improve communication.

FURTHER READING

Hurley, J. and Linsley, P. (2012) *Emotional Intelligence in Health and Social Care: a guide for improving human relationships.* CRC Press.

Motschnig, R. and Nykl, L. (2014) *Person-Centred Communication: theory, skills and practice.* Open University Press.

Rolfe, G. and Freshwater, D. (2010) *Critical Reflection in Practice: generating knowledge for care,* 2nd edition. Palgrave.

REFERENCES

Borton, T. (1970) *Reach, Teach and Touch.* McGraw-Hill.

Boud, D. (2010) Relocating reflection in the context of practice. In: Bradbury, H., Frost, N., Kilminster, S. and Zukas, M. (eds) *Beyond Reflective Practice: new approaches to professional lifelong learning.* Routledge, pp. 25–36.

Burbach, B., Barnason, S. and Thompson, S. (2015) Using 'think aloud' to capture clinical reasoning during patient simulation. *International Journal of Nursing Education and Scholarship,* **12(1)**: 1–7.

Department of Health and Social Care (2015) *The NHS Constitution for England.* Available at: www.gov.uk/government/publications/the-nhs-constitution-for-england/the-nhs-constitution-for-england (accessed 19 July 2019).

Escuriex, B. and Labbé, E. (2012) Health care providers' mindfulness and treatment outcomes: a critical review of the research literature. *Mindfulness,* **2(4)**: 242–53.

Foureur, M., Besley, K., Burton, G., Yu, N. and Crisp, J. (2013) Enhancing the resilience of nurses and midwives: pilot of a mindfulness based program for increased health, sense of coherence and decreased depression, anxiety and stress. *Contemporary Nurse,* **45(1)**: 114–25.

Francis, R. (chair) (2013) *Report of the Mid Staffordshire NHS Foundation Trust Public Inquiry.* The Stationery Office. Available at: https://assets.publishing.service.gov.uk/government/uploads/system/uploads/attachment_data/file/279124/0947.pdf (accessed 19 July 2019).

Gault, I., Shapcott, J., Luthi, A. and Reid, G. (2017) *Communication in Nursing and Healthcare: a guide for compassionate practice.* Sage.

Gibbs, G. (1988) *Learning by Doing: a guide to teaching and learning methods.* Further Education Unit, Oxford Polytechnic.

Goleman, G. (1996) *Emotional Intelligence: why it can matter more than IQ.* Bloomsbury.

NHS England (2016) *Leading Change, Adding Value: a framework for nursing, midwifery and care staff.* Available at: www.england.nhs.uk/wp-content/uploads/2016/05/nursing-framework.pdf (accessed 19 July 2019).

Nursing and Midwifery Council (2018a) *The Code: professional standards of practice and behaviour for nurses, midwives and nursing associates.* NMC. Available at: www.nmc.org.uk/globalassets/sitedocuments/nmc-publications/nmc-code.pdf (accessed 19 July 2019).

Nursing and Midwifery Council (2018b) *Future Nurse: standards of proficiency for registered nurses.* NMC. Available at: www.nmc.org.uk/globalassets/sitedocuments/education-standards/future-nurse-proficiencies.pdf (accessed 19 July 2019).

Oelofsen, N. (2012) *Developing Reflective Practice: a guide for students and practitioners of health and social care.* Lantern Publishing Ltd.

Parliamentary and Health Service Ombudsman (2011) *Care and compassion? Report of the Health Service Ombudsman on ten investigations into NHS care of older people.* Available at: www.ombudsman.org.uk/sites/default/files/2016-10/Care%20and%20Compassion.pdf (accessed 19 July 2019).

Reader, T., Gillespie, A. and Roberts, J. (2014) Patient complaints in healthcare systems: a systematic review and coding taxonomy. *British Medical Journal*, **23(8)**: 678–89.

Savage, M. (2013) Communicating with haematology patients: a reflective account. *Nursing Standard*, **28(4)**: 37–43.

Schön, D. (1983) *The Reflective Practitioner.* Basic Books.

Shannon, C. and Weaver, W. (1949) *The Mathematical Theory of Communications.* University of Illinois Press.

Snowden, A., Stenhouse, R., Young, J., Carver, H., Carver, F. and Brown, N. (2015) The relationship between emotional intelligence, previous caring experience and mindfulness in student nurses and midwives: a cross sectional analysis. *Nurse Education Today*, **35(1)**: 152–8.

Sumner, J. (2010) Reflection and moral maturity in a nurse's caring practice: a critical perspective. *Nursing Philosophy*, **11:** 159–69.

Tanner, C.A. (2006) Thinking like a nurse: a research-based model of clinical judgment in nursing. *Journal of Nursing Education*, **45**: 204–11.

van der Riet, P., Rossiter, R., Kirby, D., Dluzewska, T. and Harmon, C. (2014) Piloting a stress management and mindfulness program for undergraduate nursing students: student feedback and lessons learned. *Nurse Education Today*, **35(1)**: 44–9.

Walker, M. and Mann, R.A. (2015) Exploration of mindfulness in relation to compassion, empathy and reflection within nursing education. *Nurse Education Today*, **40**: 188–90.

Wood, J.T. (2004) *Communication Theories in Action: an introduction.* Wadsworth/Thomson Learning.

Chapter 2

Communication skills in assessing, planning, providing and managing care

Pádraig Ó Lúanaigh

LEARNING OUTCOMES

By the end of this chapter you should be able to:

2.1 Explain and apply verbal and non-verbal communication skills when assessing client and patient needs

2.2 Apply active listening skills and effective questioning to provide safe and high-quality nursing care

2.3 Use different strategies such as Caring Conversations, SBAR and Brief Intervention in your everyday practice

2.4 Understand and apply best practice principles in terms of recording and communicating your practice.

2.1 Introduction

This chapter builds on the content covered in *Chapter 1* and specifically explores the communication attributes and skills needed to assess, plan, provide and manage the care you and nursing colleagues provide. The content presented will challenge you to consider and think about the theories and concepts of communication and how you can apply this knowledge directly to your clinical practice. You will have an opportunity in this chapter to reflect on your existing communication skills and start to think about how effective and professional communication will support you to provide safe, quality nursing care.

The central focus of this chapter draws on the UK Nursing and Midwifery Council's *Future Nurse: standards of proficiency for registered nurses* and the reference to the importance of effective communication:

> .... *because a diverse range of communication and relationship management skills is required to ensure that individuals, their families and carers are actively involved in*

and understand care decisions. These skills are vital when making accurate, culturally aware assessments of care needs and ensuring that the needs, priorities, expertise and preferences of people are always valued and taken into account.

(Nursing and Midwifery Council, 2018a, p. 27)

This quote reflects the essence of quality nursing care and the achievement of true person-centred care. While you will read about communication in this book, it is vital to recognise that your own self-awareness and personal qualities play just as important a part in your effective professional communication.

Effective communication takes practice and there will be times throughout your career when interactions and your intended outcome do not go the way you planned. To be a confident professional communicator you will need to be brave, to take risks and use feedback from others, supported by personal reflection. This chapter provides references to online media examples and activities that will encourage you to engage with issues you will encounter in your nursing practice. You may be surprised to discover you already have many of the skills your professional life requires! The next section looks at verbal and non-verbal communication skills from a nursing perspective and lays the foundation for the techniques and frameworks which are presented later in this chapter.

2.2 Verbal and non-verbal communication

When considering the types of communication skills used in working with clients and patient groups it is interesting to reflect on how much of what you communicate, and is communicated to you, is not actually spoken. Very often it is the unspoken that will provide important information and help you in your assessment and decision-making. Verbal and non-verbal communication go hand in hand and both should be seen as essential in ensuring an effective communication episode.

Equally, when considering how to enable person-centred and individualised care – and not appearing as the 'know it all' professional – remember that the words 'listen' and 'silent' are spelt using the same letters. It is important to make this point because, as professional care providers, we often fail to listen and can be fearful of allowing silence in our interactions with individuals.

Your non-verbal actions and practice can communicate very powerful negative and uncaring attitudes. At times, we forget that a 'throw away' comment or failure to smile or acknowledge can convey very negative messages. Think of the times you have felt ignored in a shop or where the staff have engaged in a private conversation while leaving you to wait. Have you ever observed clinical staff who are using a computer or writing notes at a nurse's station, completely oblivious of a patient or their relative standing waiting to speak to them?

Think about how you stand, and the hand gestures or facial expressions you use when speaking to individuals and the messages these convey without you ever having to speak. Remember in your assessment activities that there will be many factors influencing communication, affecting both yourself and the patient. The list below is an example of these but can you think of others?

- Personal values
- Personal space
- Environment
- Awareness
- Perceptions
- Social and cultural background
- Knowledge and understanding
- Language
- Role and relationships
- Emotions

The SOLER model shown in *Table 2.1* has been used to good effect in promoting the 'listener' as a fundamental part of the conversation relationship, and was introduced in 1975 by Gerard Egan, an American psychologist. He referred to 'micro skills', which we can adopt as part of a therapeutic relationship. Using this model encourages active listening through non-verbal approaches, which is useful in holistic assessment (Stickley, 2011).

Table 2.1 *The SOLER model*

Sit squarely	Sit directly opposite the patient where applicable, although some may feel this is a little threatening. Egan acknowledges that positioning may need to be altered, but in general terms, you should face the patient.
Open posture	This is recommended to avoid aggressive or perceived barriers to honest conversations. Egan suggests sitting with arms and hands relaxed in your lap or at your side, not crossed. Legs and feet should not be crossed.
Lean towards the other	Egan suggests this stance can help the patient see you are interested in what they are saying. However, you must respect personal space and not lean forward in a way that can seem intimidating. A nod of the head when the patient is speaking will reaffirm you are listening and hearing what is being said. Although not specifically 'non-verbal', an 'umm' occasionally during a conversation can also reinforce this.
Eye contact	Maintaining eye contact is important in all communication activities. In non-verbal communication, this shows you are interested and focused on what the individual is saying. Do not look at your watch, the clock on the wall, or out of the window. This will make you appear rushed, distracted or uninterested. Be aware of cultural sensitivities relating to eye contact.
Relax	This relates to the listener being calm and relaxed, not fidgeting or appearing nervous. A relaxed manner can help to build a trusting relationship with your patient by instilling confidence.

A criticism of the SOLER approach is the lack of reference to facial expression and touch. Research has shown that many non-verbal communication methods such as social touch, eye contact and a smile, have an impact on how patients view a clinician's empathy (Montague *et al.*, 2013). Facial expressions are an important part of developing and building a relationship. A beaming smile when meeting bereaved relatives is not appropriate, so you must assess each situation and adapt your expressions and body language accordingly. Non-verbal communication is about being self-aware and thinking about the situation presented to you. Be prepared to watch other role models and practise methods with your supervisor. Ask for feedback, as you may not realise how you are perceived by others.

Ali (2017) suggests it is vital that nurses see the patient behind the task throughout any activity. It is often reported that nurses will introduce themselves and explain they need to conduct an assessment activity such as taking a temperature, although the reading is rarely given to the patient. Consider whether this could reassure the patient, if the reading is within normal limits, or could help to build a trusting relationship if you discuss that the reading is above normal limits, explaining why this could be the case and what actions you will take to monitor this/refer onwards. It is important you check for understanding because we can all have selective hearing to some extent, choosing to retain information we see as important. Accepting a verbal 'yes I understand' from a patient does not always mean they do understand. Ask them to explain it back to you if this is appropriate, or check for facial expressions when you are giving an explanation. Do they look confused? If so, amend your explanation in simple terms.

Many authors suggest that both patients and healthcare staff's satisfaction rates increase when communication is honest, transparent and understood (Ennis *et al.*, 2013; Groves, 2014; Pines *et al.*, 2012). Therefore, always think of the variety of communication methods at your disposal to ensure your message is conveyed and understood, with a willingness to accept that this may need to be adapted during the process.

An important aspect of any verbal communication to consider is not only the words used, but the tone or manner in which they are spoken. Two key points you should adopt when communicating verbally are:
- Be clear, honest and accurate.
- Ensure appropriateness to age, language, culture and level of understanding.

How people interpret what you say will depend on how you say it. This includes the pitch of your voice, as well as the volume, emphasis and pace. If you're asking a patient questions in a cold, stern manner, they are unlikely to respond with their true feelings. They may feel you are hurried or perceive you as someone who is harsh and uncaring. This can have negative consequences in building a trusting relationship, with the patient unlikely to divulge information that could be important to their treatment and care. Be aware of how loud or quiet your natural tone is and remember to adapt this sensitively to suit the situation. For example, do not think someone who has difficulty in hearing needs you to shout, as this can be embarrassing for the patient and may not improve their hearing or understanding of your words. Clearly spoken sentences, directly in front of the patient, may be a more appropriate method.

ACTIVITY 2.1

A. Watch 'Caring Conversations – Craig's Story': https://tinyurl.com/yaklncod
- What did you identify from the actions of Craig's GP that had an impact on his consultation?
- What were the verbal and non-verbal messages that were conveyed to Craig?
- What could have been done differently to improve this interaction?
- How will your clinical practice change because of watching this video?

B. Now please watch 'Caring Conversations – John's Film': https://tinyurl.com/ycj4nvfj
- John describes how a member of staff treated him differently – what were the actions by the member of staff which John described?
- Have you ever been aware of your attitude changing towards a patient based on information about them?
- Are you aware of your own behaviour changing after hearing information about someone (for example 'infectious patient', 'came with police escort', 'rough sleeper', 'has dementia', 'can be violent' or 'used to be a nurse')?

C. Finally, now watch 'Caring Conversations – Joy's Story': https://tinyurl.com/y8ce9z7n
- How was Joy supported by the other character and encouraged to explain her experience (look for the non-verbal actions)?
- How would you have continued the conversation if Joy was describing an experience of where you were working as a registered nurse?
- Do you think the nurse in this scenario was 'nasty' or was it an 'accident'/poor communication?

Thinking about the three patient experiences, there were examples of prejudice, poor communication, and failing to treat the person as an individual, and while very little was verbally said the patients each identified very strong non-verbal messages. The theme common across the three examples was of patients not being 'treated as a human being'.

2.3 Active listening and appropriate questioning

This section will describe some approaches you can use to ask questions that support your assessment and therapeutic communication with your patients. There is no need to 'learn' tricks or ways to demonstrate or convey that you are paying attention and interested in someone – people know if you are genuine and interested in what they're saying, if you're actually paying attention and listening to them!

It can be challenging to support patients to explain how they feel or have the confidence to ask questions that enable the individual to articulate clearly. One technique you can use is envision cards, which can be used in different ways to support people to describe an experience, feeling or story using a trigger word or image. The cards provide an alternative approach that does not depend on your asking a series of questions, which may feel intimidating or leading. You can download a useful set of envision cards from: https://nes.scot.nhs.uk/education-and-training/by-discipline/nursing-and-midwifery/resources/publications/valuing-feedback-envision-cards.aspx

Download the cards and test their usefulness by asking someone you know to select a picture or word card that sums up how they feel about working in a clinical area, learning on a course, or being cared for in hospital, or ask them to select a card that best reflects their emotional state and that sums up for them what different experiences feel like. Reflect on the discussion and how useful this approach was. Did the approach allow the other person to be more in control of the conversation and did it allow and encourage them to describe and communicate their feelings, experiences or emotions more clearly? Did the conversation provide you with a better understanding and insight into what the other person wanted to say?

The use of such trigger images or words can be a useful way of engaging and starting a conversation with individuals of all ages and needs.

As you consider how you communicate with patients, colleagues and families in your professional role, it is important to remember that the most effective communication will be when you are authentic. Every individual and client group will require and challenge you to consider how you communicate. Consider how your communication style and approach would need to adapt when interacting with individuals with a learning disability, children, those who are deaf or blind or who do not speak your language. As you develop your skills, make use of simple phrases and practise using open and closed questions. As a general rule, closed questions will require a 'yes' or 'no' answer, while open questions require more than a one-word answer and a more in-depth response. They usually include 'how', 'what' and 'why' questions. Some examples of these are shown below. Try not to use judgemental language or use your opinions or past experiences when talking with patients – don't equate your experience with theirs (all experiences are individual). Most importantly don't expect to always have the answer, if you don't know – say you don't know, and remember silence and listening is fine.

Closed questions	Open questions
Are you feeling better today?	How are you feeling today?
Do you need help?	How I can help you?
Are you in pain?	Can you describe how your pain is today?
Would you like to sit up?	How can I make your position more comfortable for you?
Are you thirsty/hungry?	Can you tell me why you don't want to eat and drink today?

2.3.1 This is me

Individuals with dementia need skilled and compassionate care based on informed and appropriate communication skills. 'This is me' is a widely used and useful resource which you can use in your practice. The document is a useful resource in knowing individuals with dementia better and can support you in providing individualised care. You can download a copy from: www.alzheimers.org.uk/get-support/publications-factsheets/this-is-me

Read the document and think about the kinds of questions/areas covered. Consider how having this completed document could support your nursing care of a patient. Are there areas of information in this form that you could incorporate into your assessments and conversations with patients? You may have seen this document used in practice areas. If you have, ask carers and family members how beneficial they find the form to support care of their relative.

You will find further discussion of communication strategies relating to communication vulnerability in *Chapter 5*.

ACTIVITY 2.2

Watch the following two short videos of healthcare staff talking about their interactions with patients:

https://tinyurl.com/y9n7pdxe and https://tinyurl.com/y9mvuk74

- The first speaker talks about "being in the patient's skin" to practise and communicate effectively. Reflect on a patient you can recall and try to see your interaction from the patient's perspective (be in their skin). How do you think they really perceived you?
- Think about how you communicated and interacted with that patient – would you do anything differently if you had the opportunity to repeat the interaction?
- The second speaker, Jacqui, described an interaction she had with one of her clients. What did you think about how she communicated with the patient?
- Think about the ways that you communicate – how will you ensure that you're able to communicate in a way that meets the needs of everyone?

2.4 Emotional vocabulary

Previously you considered the use of envision cards and how these can be used to encourage and support individuals to talk about their experiences and feelings. There is also a need for you to develop and make use of an effective emotional vocabulary to be able to elicit accurate and relevant information from those you are caring for. There is a useful online resource at: www.caringconversations.scot/sites/default/files/emotional_vocabulary_a4_0.pdf

The web resource provides a list of words that you can use in your conversations and questions with patients. The words are reproduced in *Activity 2.3* below, which is designed to support you to practise using these words.

ACTIVITY 2.3

The following list of emotional words can be used in asking questions and to support more detailed and accurate assessments.

Read through the list of words and phrases now.

At ease	Calm	Cheerful	Comfortable
Comforted	Confident	Excited	Fortunate
Happy	Heard	Hopeful	In control
Included	Moved	Optimistic	Over the moon
Positive	Protected	Proud	Privileged
Reassured	Relieved	Respected	Safe
Satisfied	Supported	Welcomed	
Alarmed	Anxious	Awful	Awkward
Brushed off	Cagey	Cut off	Defensive
Dejected	Disheartened	Dismissed	Dreadful
Fed up	Flustered	Frustrated	Intimidated
Let down	Messed about	Rushed	Shocked
Nervous	Scared	Sorry	Shaken
Uncomfortable	Upset		

Did you recognise all the words? If there are any you don't understand, search for their definition.

- Which words do you use in your daily conversations?
- Are there any you rarely or never currently use?
- Think about an event/experience in your life. Try to use at least five of the words in the emotional vocabulary list to describe how the event made you feel as you describe the experience.
- Did the words you used help in better capturing and reflecting how you *felt* during the experience?

2.5 Caring conversations

This section of the chapter takes what you have learnt, reflected on and discovered in the previous section and looks to build this into your developing ability to have caring conversations.

Before exploring what caring conversations are, establishing any conversation at the outset is extremely important and this seems a natural time to mention the *#hello my name is* campaign. There is an online resource where the late Dr Kate Granger describes why she started the campaign based on her experience as a patient and her awareness of the failure of healthcare staff to introduce themselves (see www.youtube.com/watch?v=UmeQjgy4QnE).

#hello my name is has been widely adopted across health systems and you may have seen this in use during your placements. Even if the campaign is not formally implemented there is nothing to stop you adopting this practice by introducing yourself: "Hello my name is … and I am a …. and I would like to assist/help/give you … if that is OK?"

It is also important to think about shaking your patient's hand when you meet and/or conclude your interaction with them if you feel the situation is appropriate – do not underestimate the power of touch. The Caring Conversations framework (Dewar and Nolan, 2013) aims to enhance the way we engage with each other and thereby to support the provision of compassionate care. Caring Conversations provides guidance on having meaningful dialogue and is a useful approach to practise as you gain confidence in having conversations with patients. There are seven Cs that structure having caring conversations (http://myhomelife. org.uk/our-guiding-principles/having-caring-conversations/#main):

- **Being Courageous** (What matters? What would happen if we gave this a go? What is the worst that could happen if you did this?)
- **Connecting emotionally** (How did this make you feel?)
- **Being Curious** (What strikes you about this? What prompted you to act in this way? What helped this to happen?)
- **Collaboration** (How can we work together to make this happen? What do you need to do to make this happen?)
- **Considering other perspectives** (Help me to understand where you are coming from? What do others think? What is real and possible? What might the other person be thinking?)
- **Compromising** (What is important to you? What would you like to happen?)
- **Celebrating** (What worked well here? Why did it work well? How can we help this to happen more of the time? What are our strengths in being able to achieve this?)

Each of the elements above builds on the earlier content in this chapter and provides open question examples that you can use. Initially you may not be able to incorporate all seven elements into your conversation. However, the structure and examples will provide you with some useful trigger questions and structure to ensure you have meaningful and effective questions to gather appropriate information. This will in turn help to inform your nursing assessment and promote therapeutic conversations with your patients.

ACTIVITY 2.4

Watch Angie's story: https://tinyurl.com/y8xwwhr7

Consider the different experiences Angie had with her various GPs.
- If you were caring for Angie what questions would you ask her based on the Caring Conversations seven Cs?
- Near the end, listen to the description Angie gave of a GP she had a good relationship with. What words did she use to describe him?
- Think about how this GP reassured Angie in relation to his own lifestyle – can you identify examples of some of the Caring Conversations framework in how he engaged with Angie?

2.6 Brief Intervention

Brief Intervention is an established way of engaging with patients and is used as part of the approach in promoting health and the Making Every Contact Count (MECC) campaign.

Brief Intervention will seem like Caring Conversations in structure in that again it is structured, this time around five As. The following example demonstrates how you would use the five As to support an individual who was a smoker (www.hse.ie/eng/about/who/tobaccocontrol/intervention/):
- **Ask**: systematically identify all smokers at every visit. Record smoking status, number of cigarettes smoked per day/week and year started smoking.
- **Advise**: urge all smokers to quit. Advice should be clear and personalised.
- **Assess**: determine willingness and confidence to make a quit attempt.
- **Assist**: aid the smoker in quitting. Provide behavioural support. Recommend/prescribe pharmacological aids. If not ready to quit, promote motivation for future attempt.
- **Arrange**: follow-up appointment within 1 week or if appropriate refer to specialist cessation service for intensive support. Document the intervention.

Brief Intervention is designed to be exactly that – a structured way to engage with patients as part of routine contact to explore and support lifestyle and behaviour change. This approach provides you with another structured approach to your interactions and conversations with patients which is focused on supporting their health and wellbeing. Your interactions with clients and patients should always be focused and purposeful, and your interactions should inform your nursing assessment and evaluation of care – they should never be merely 'chats'.

Making Every Contact Count (MECC) and Brief Intervention are discussed further in *Chapter 3*.

2.7 **Duty of candour**

Finally, this section will highlight the importance of disclosure or the duty of candour as an essential component of authentic and professional interactions with the public. The duty of candour is the foundation of an honest and trusting relationship between you and your patients. The requirement it places on you is that you will always be open and honest when there has been an incident or mistake in relation to care. You must always be prepared to provide full and accurate explanations to your patients about the care you provide and explain any mistakes and apologise for these.

ACTIVITY 2.5

Please watch this short video about duty of candour:

www.youtube.com/watch?v=ccnlhxa60w8

What do you think the key message was in the film?
- Find out what the process is in your current placement in terms of recording incidents and how duty of candour is achieved.
- How is learning from incidents shared in the organisation you are currently based in?
- Read the NMC guidance on duty of candour here: www.nmc.org.uk/standards/guidance/the-professional-duty-of-candour/read-the-professional-duty-of-candour/

Glasper (2015) suggests that nursing staff may be unsure whether a particular situation should be raised as a concern. You can always refer to the raising concerns guidance from your education institute or organisation for additional information. The most important thing to remember is not to ignore it! Speak with the senior clinician or team member for the area, as NMC guidance requires someone in the team to take responsibility. Sharing learning from these episodes can be very powerful, encouraging transparency and promoting a learning culture within the workplace.

2.8 **Written communication**

Your professional communication and documentation will be captured in a range of ways, such as your written nursing documentation, in emails, on the telephone, text messages or other electronic communication portals.

Guidance on the maintenance of your nursing records is provided in the NMC's *Code* (Nursing and Midwifery Council, 2018b). The guidance in Section 10 of the *Code* is reproduced below for your information.

NMC CODE SECTION 10

Keep clear and accurate records relevant to your practice.

This applies to the records that are relevant to your scope of practice. It includes but is not limited to patient records.

To achieve this, you must:

10.1 complete records at the time or as soon as possible after an event, recording if the notes are written some time after the event

10.2 identify any risks or problems that have arisen and the steps taken to deal with them, so that colleagues who use the records have all the information they need

10.3 complete records accurately and without any falsification, taking immediate and appropriate action if you become aware that someone has not kept to these requirements

10.4 attribute any entries you make in any paper or electronic records to yourself, making sure they are clearly written, dated and timed, and do not include unnecessary abbreviations, jargon or speculation

10.5 take all steps to make sure that records are kept securely

10.6 collect, treat and store all data and research findings appropriately

This NMC guidance is applicable regardless of how you record your practice, whether on paper, in electronic records or in emails.

- Your documentation entries should always be dated and timed.
- Keep your format consistent and clear throughout.
- When recording times, the 24-hour clock format is preferable but regardless do not switch between or mix formats (3.00pm and 18:00hrs, for example).
- Avoid the use of uncommon abbreviations where possible.
- Handwriting should be clear and legible.
- Always sign all entries and print your name and designation.
- Use clear, simple language to present facts, avoiding personal opinions.

Fowler (2014) highlights the growing number of cases reported to the NMC regarding poor record-keeping. These include making false entries, not maintaining adequate records (such as a risk or pain assessment), stating that certain processes/activities had taken place when they had not. Therefore, we must value and acknowledge the importance of good written communication to ensure consistency and accuracy of care. It is also important to give feedback to your colleagues if you feel their written notes and feedback are difficult to understand, or are not in the required depth and breadth to effectively continue seamless patient care. Learning from each other can influence positive ways of improving practice and sharing ideas.

ACTIVITY 2.6

Review one of your recent patient records and an entry you have made. Assess your entry and those of colleagues against the following:

- Is there an accurate assessment of the person's physical, psychological and social wellbeing and, whenever necessary, the views and observations of family members in relation to that assessment?
- Is there evidence of decision-making and care delivery by nurses and midwives?
- Is there an evaluation of the effectiveness, or otherwise, of the nursing/midwifery care provided?

Taken from the *Nursing and Midwifery Board of Ireland – Recording Clinical Practice Guidelines* www.nmbi.ie/nmbi/media/NMBI/Publications/recording-clinical-practice-professional-guidance.pdf?ext=.pdf

Locate the policy in your placement area related to documentation and read the guidance and local policies in relation to documentation.

2.9 **Social media and electronic communication**

We're all familiar with the benefits and use of social media. However, in a professional care context you need to view and treat social media and electronic communication with a different approach to how you communicate in your personal life. As a regulated professional and employee, there are expectations on your behaviour and actions which are informed by legal considerations (freedom of information, confidentiality), professional considerations (codes of conduct) and employment considerations (dignity and harassment at work policies) included for example.

The fundamental consideration in terms of social media is patient confidentiality and the absolute need for you to ensure that you do not breach a patient's right to confidentiality or allow them to be identified because of any written communication or image you may post online.

You must also be alert to any comment or image that may call into question your professional integrity. Equally, you need to manage your publicly visible profiles and social media accounts in terms of the potential to receive 'friend' or follower requests from current or ex-patients. Such social media connections can create the potential for very difficult issues in relation to maintaining professional boundaries.

The NMC also has specific guidance relating to the use of social media and this should be used in conjunction with the *Code* (www.nmc.org.uk/standards/guidance/social-media-guidance/).

The *Code*, paragraph 20.10, states: "Use all forms of spoken, written and digital communication (including social media and networking sites) responsibly." The web link above states that a qualified nurse's registration may be at risk and student nurses risk not being able to join the NMC register if they act in any way that is unprofessional or unlawful on social media, including:

- sharing confidential information inappropriately
- posting pictures of patients and people receiving care without their consent
- posting inappropriate comments about patients
- bullying, intimidating or exploiting people
- building or pursuing relationships with patients or service users
- stealing personal information or using someone else's identity
- encouraging violence or self-harm
- inciting hatred or discrimination.

Nevertheless, electronic communication can be very effective in providing patient support. Wagg *et al.* (2018) completed a systematic literature review looking at the effectiveness of computer-mediated communication, which included teleconferencing, Facebook forums, YouTube and email. The review suggested 81% of the studies reviewed indicated a positive benefit of media communication to provide patient support and were valued by patients. As communication technology advances, and resources continue to be scrutinised, this is an important area to embrace in future nursing and healthcare provision. There are obvious pitfalls, with easy access to electronic platforms that provide non-evidence-based health information. This can be challenging when conducting assessments if patients already have a preconceived idea of their condition/treatment from a questionable source of information. However, Risling *et al.* (2017) suggest that we need to explore this medium further to maximise its potential in nursing practice and have produced a social media assessment tool and associated assessment package for family nursing in Canada. Engagement of specific groups who do not always access healthcare services, such as adolescents, can be successfully achieved through social media communication.

2.10 Sharing information effectively

A key element of your nursing care is the effective sharing and communication with colleagues directly and indirectly who are also involved with providing input to your patients. Your care record is an essential element of demonstrating the nursing input that was provided and provides a long-term account of the care provided.

This next section will explore ways of providing a clinical handover of care and the key elements of best practice in terms of documenting your care. An aspect of nursing practice that can provoke some anxiety in junior staff is providing a concise yet comprehensive verbal clinical handover to colleagues. You may have already had experience of handovers that seemed to consist of abbreviations and at the end you were still unclear about what care was provided, or the plan of care for the patient.

One framework which is widely used and provides a useful way to structure your sharing of information and clinical handover is called SBAR. The letters stand for:

- S = Situation (a concise statement of the problem)
- B = Background (pertinent and brief information related to the situation)

- A = Assessment (analysis and considerations of options — what you found/think)
- R = Recommendation (action requested/recommended — what you want)

The SBAR approach can be used in any clinical situation. When used appropriately, it provides a simple structure to focus reporting in a way that allows you to articulate, and those listening to understand, the current and intended plan of care for the patient.

ACTIVITY 2.7

Recall a patient you have cared for recently or a clinical handover which you feel could have been better structured.

Using the information you can remember, write down what you could have said using the SBAR format.

- Did you find it easy to provide information for each section of the SBAR?
- Frequently we spend a lot of time describing the Situation and Background but the Assessment and Recommendations are much harder to discuss. If this was your experience, why do you think we find the Situation and Background easier to do?
- If SBAR is not used in your clinical area, ask colleagues whether they have used this approach and what format they use to structure their clinical handovers.

The final part of this chapter focuses on a case study, which will support you to consider the ideas covered and practise all the elements you have worked through. If possible speak with a colleague to share your ideas about the case study. Discuss your approaches, considering possible similarities and differences in your and your colleague's approaches to dealing with the activity.

CASE STUDY

You have just arrived at your clinical area to start your shift. As you walk into the bay of patients you will be responsible for, the registered nurse handing over says: "We've had a busy morning, bed seven should have gone by now, but her family haven't turned up yet."

As you start to receive your handover the hospital porters arrive with a patient for admission. The patient is an older adult who appears distressed. The nurse in charge says: "She was supposed to go in there – to bed seven – but we have nowhere to put her yet. The other one's family haven't turned up to take her."

The porter shrugs his shoulders and says: "So what do you want me to do with this one?"
- How could this situation be managed?
- Consider the range of communication skills you will need to reassure your patient(s) in this situation, your nursing colleague and the porter.
- What would you say and do?

The family of the patient for discharge arrive and apologise profusely but they could not find anywhere to park and spent 30 minutes waiting for a space. They then went to the wrong ward.

CASE STUDY (*continued*)

You start to admit your new patient and due to the circumstances realise you didn't get any clinical handover so review the notes that were provided. There is very little documented other than 'admitted from nursing home following a fall, appears confused and ?? dementia'.

- Think about how you will approach this patient and how you will initiate the conversation.
- What would you do to gain trust and reassure this patient?
- The patient appears a little disorientated but not confused. Think about the words and language you would use to start assessing the patient's needs.

It becomes apparent that the patient has full recall of her situation and she receives treatment for a urinary tract infection and a review of her medication.

- Think about how you would provide a clinical handover to the next staff on duty. Consider the situation from this patient's initial arrival on the ward, to the care you provided during the shift, and the framework you could use to do so.
- You decide to discuss the experience with your ward manager and the issues around not having a bed ready for your new patient. Your manager asks you to write a statement because they were concerned by the poor level of communication you describe and wants to raise the matter with your colleague. Write a short statement detailing the events that occurred during the handover for your manager.

Summary

This chapter has encouraged you to think about what is different when communicating professionally and the skills you need to assess, plan and communicate your nursing care. Professional communication is multifaceted and reflects complexities in nursing practice. Over time you will develop your own nursing 'voice' and this will progress if you are willing to practise different approaches and engage with colleagues to seek feedback on how to improve your communication. Make use of any opportunity to observe and listen to your colleagues and learn from how they communicate verbally and non-verbally. Remember to reflect on the good interactions and what worked with patients and of course the times when things do not go as you had intended. Practise and perfect your nursing documentation and clinical handover skills, making a commitment to yourself to always maintain NMC standards, regardless of how busy, tired or unconfident you feel. If things go wrong, always report them. Finally, remember to provide feedback to your colleagues on their communication, be brave and acknowledge the good, but also be ready to challenge any poor communication you witness.

KEY LEARNING POINTS

Four key points to take away from *Chapter 2*:

- ☑ Effective communication is complex and draws on both verbal and non-verbal forms of communication.
- ☑ There are numerous frameworks and approaches to support your development as a good communicator in assessing and planning care.
- ☑ Caring conversations take time and practice to perfect. Learn from colleagues as role models.
- ☑ Careful attention must be paid to how you document and communicate your assessments, plan of care and records of care.

FURTHER READING AND RESOURCES

#hello my name is: www.hellomynameis.org.uk/

Institute for Healthcare Improvement. SBAR Tool: Situation-Background-Assessment-Recommendation: www.ihi.org/resources/Pages/Tools/SBARToolkit.aspx

NHS Health Education England. Making Every Contact Count: www.makingeverycontactcount.com/

Nursing and Midwifery Board of Ireland. Recording Clinical Practice: www.nmbi.ie/nmbi/media/NMBI/Publications/recording-clinical-practice-professional-guidance.pdf?ext=.pdf

Nursing and Midwifery Board of Ireland. Guidance to Nurses and Midwives on Social Media and Social Networking: www.nmbi.ie/nmbi/media/NMBI/Publications/Guidance-to-Nurses-Midwives-on-Social-Media-Social-Networking.pdf?ext=.pdf

Waverley Care. Putting Caring Conversations into Practice: www.caringconversations.scot/

REFERENCES

Ali, M. (2017) Communication skills 1: benefits of effective communication for patients. *Nursing Times*, **113(12)**: 18–19.

Dewar, B. and Nolan, M. (2013) Caring about caring: developing a model to implement compassionate relationship centred care in an older people care setting. *International Journal of Nursing Studies*, **50(9)**: 1247–58.

Ennis, G., Happell, B., Broadbent, M. and Reid-Searl, K. (2013) The importance of communication for clinical leaders in mental health nursing: the perspective of nurses working in mental health. *Mental Health Nursing*, **34(11)**: 814–19.

Fowler, J. (2014) Written communication from staff nurse to nurse consultant. Part 2: patient records. *British Journal of Nursing*, **23(16)**: 910.

Glasper, J. (2015) The professional duty of candour. *British Journal of Nursing*, **24(16)**: 840–1.

Groves, W. (2014) Professional practice skills for nurses. *Nursing Standard*, **29(1)**: 51–9.

Montague, E., Chen, P., Xu, J., Chewning, B. and Barrett, B. (2013) Nonverbal interpersonal interactions in clinical encounters and patient perceptions of empathy. *Journal of Participatory Medicine*, **Aug 14**: 5:e33.

Nursing and Midwifery Council (2018a) *Future Nurse: standards of proficiency for registered nurses*. NMC. Available at: www.nmc.org.uk/globalassets/ sitedocuments/education-standards/future-nurse-proficiencies.pdf (accessed 19 July 2019).

Nursing and Midwifery Council (2018b) *The Code: professional standards of practice and behaviour for nurses, midwives and nursing associates*. NMC. Available at: www.nmc.org.uk/globalassets/sitedocuments/nmc-publications/ nmc-code.pdf (accessed 19 July 2019).

Pines, E.W., Rauschhuber, M.L., Norgan, G.H., Cook, J.D., Canchola, L., Richardson, C. and Jones, M.E. (2012) Stress resiliency, psychological empowerment and conflict management styles among baccalaureate nursing students. *Journal of Advanced Nursing*, **68(7)**: 1482–93.

Risling, T., Risling, D. and Holtslander, L. (2017) Creating a social media assessment tool for family nursing. *Journal of Family Nursing*, **23(1)**: 13–33.

Stickley, T. (2011) From SOLER to SURETY for effective nonverbal communication. *Nurse Education in Practice*, **11(6)**: 395–8.

Wagg, A.J., Callanan, M. and Hassett, A. (2018) The use of computer mediated communication in providing patient support: a review of the research literature. *International Journal of Nursing Studies*, **82**: 68–78.

Chapter 3
Communication skills in promoting health

Alison Lewis

LEARNING OUTCOMES

By the end of this chapter you should be able to:

3.1 Understand the impact of effective health promotion communication strategies

3.2 Recognise the importance of motivation and behaviour change

3.3 Appreciate the need for an evidence-based approach to promoting health

3.4 Describe communication approaches that could be used to address common health risk behaviours seen in various patient/client groups.

3.1 Introduction

The communication skills required to undertake health promotion stem from the Ottawa Charter for Health Promotion (World Health Organization, 1986) definition, which states that: "Health promotion is the process of enabling people to increase control over the determinants of health."

This definition implies that there are two strands to health promotion – the process to improving health **and** empowering people to take control over their health. Whilst recognising the social determinants of health are often out of an individual's control, empowering a patient/client to take control over an aspect of their health creates a positive experience for that individual. Communication becomes the pivotal tool that health promoters must apply in order to meet these two components. Health promoters need multiple skills to undertake this work, ranging from one-to-one communication skills to more facilitative skills for group sessions. There is also an emphasis on listening and understanding how people receive and interpret information, as well as being able to assess motivation for a change in health behaviour.

This chapter will discuss some of the communication skills you can employ with your clients and patients to achieve the health promotion aspects of the Ottawa Charter, to help reinforce health messages in a positive way for the people and communities you care for.

3.2 Assessing motivation for change

As nurses, it is important we understand how motivated our patient or client is to make a health behaviour change, before offering health promotion information. The days of the healthcare professional 'telling' patients how to be healthier should now be disappearing from current healthcare communications. We now know this approach is not effective, as some of the health issues we currently see increasing have demonstrated, for example obesity or type 2 diabetes.

There are a number of models and theories we can use to ensure a robust assessment is made prior to any health promotion intervention. If you would like further information on these, you can access additional reading materials in the Further reading section of this chapter. The model we will discuss in this chapter is the 'transtheoretical model', as described by Prochaska and DiClemente in 1983 and deemed to be a seminal piece of work within this area of health promotion (see *Figure 3.1*).

The model is based on five phases of change, through which a person will move in a cyclical manner from precontemplation to maintenance, whilst recognising at all points that relapse may be inevitable through this process. It is widely agreed that relapse is part of making long-term health behaviour changes, and this model

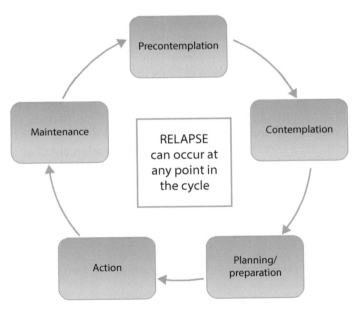

Figure 3.1 *Adapted from the transtheoretical model of behaviour change (Prochaska and DiClemente, 1983).*

encourages the nurse to help people at all stages of motivation and readiness to change, rather than just focusing on the few who are at the action phase. By listening to our patients, we can identify where they are within this model and subsequently offer appropriate guidance and discussion to help them move to the next phase.

At the precontemplation phase, an individual who smokes is not thinking about stopping smoking, whereas someone at the preparation phase is making active plans and setting a quit date. Between these two phases is contemplation, where the individual is thinking about stopping smoking and wants to make the change, but is unable to do so. It is within this phase that an individual can be helped to identify their motivation for change, as it is dependent on how important the change feels to that individual and how confident they are of achieving it. This discussion around importance and confidence is based on Bandura's (1977) theory of self-efficacy, where self-efficacy refers to an individual's belief in his or her capacity to execute behaviours necessary to produce specific performance attainments. Self-efficacy reflects a confidence in the ability to exert control over one's own motivation, behaviour and social environment. It is most useful to reflect upon in situations which trigger relapse.

During the precontemplation and contemplation phases, an individual's self-efficacy to make a change or abstain from a behaviour (i.e. how important the change in behaviour is deemed to be and level of confidence to make the change) is lower than the temptation to continue with the unhealthy behaviour. An example of this may be the patient who is within these phases and asked to discuss the benefits and drawbacks of smoking, and the benefits significantly outweigh the drawbacks.

Within the preparation and action phases, self-efficacy has increased to a point where the gap between wanting to make a change and temptation to continue with unhealthy behaviour has narrowed and the patient is able to make a healthy change.

Finally, when relapse occurs, temptation has overpowered an individual's self-efficacy, and they thus adopt the unhealthy behaviour once more. This stage is very important in the model of change, as in the case of smoking, it is recognised that an individual will relapse on average three times before they are able to stop smoking permanently (Table 3.1).

Another factor to consider when assessing motivation for change in our patients is how health literate the individual is. The World Health Organization, at their 9th Global Conference on Health Promotion in Shanghai (WHO, 2017), defined health literacy as: "the cognitive and social skills which determine the motivation and ability of individuals to gain access to, understand and use information in ways that promote and maintain good health".

In order to move from the precontemplative to the contemplative phase of the transtheoretical model, a patient requires some degree of health knowledge and understanding. As a nurse working with an individual in this phase, a discussion around what information they would like and what they already know is vital.

Table 3.1 *Summary of the stages of behaviour change*

Precontemplation	The individual is not actively thinking about changing their behaviour but may become aware that change is desirable. The nurse may be able to help move an individual to the contemplation stage by asking open questions such as "How are you feeling about your health?"
Contemplation	The individual becomes clear that change is needed and may start to research possible means to achieve the desired change. The nurse will be able to help identify their motivation for change and may enhance their confidence and self-efficacy. A discussion of the benefits and drawbacks of making the change may be helpful.
Planning	The individual is actively developing a plan of how they will implement the change. The nurse can support this stage by providing information requested by the individual (see below).
Action	The individual's desire to make the change is now stronger than the temptation to continue as they are and they take action such as actively accessing health services, joining a support group, etc.
Maintenance	The individual takes steps to ensure that the change is lasting.
Relapse	This can occur at any stage in the change process – for example an individual trying to quit smoking will relapse on average three times before stopping permanently. At this stage a discussion of the individual's self-efficacy may support them to attempt to change again.

The 'Elicit–Provide–Elicit' technique from motivational interviewing (Miller and Rollnick, 2012) is an appropriate approach to use. This requires the health professional to ask:

- what the individual already knows about the issue
- how they feel about making a change
- what information they would like from the nurse to help them move into the planning phase.

(See *Chapter 4* for more information about motivational interviewing.)

The nurse can then provide the individual with the information requested (and in the format requested by the person) in a non-judgemental and supportive manner. This will ultimately increase the individual's health literacy regarding the behaviour change they wish to make and help them to feel in control of their own health and lifestyle. The nurse then ensures that the patient has all the information they need and can assess how ready they are to change.

It is also important when assessing motivation for change that there is 'congruence' between nurse and patient. Congruence occurs when the conversation that you are having with your patient is aligned to their thoughts and feelings about the desire to make health behavioural changes. If it is not, you may face resistance from your patient and possible return to a previous phase of the model.

The following scenario illustrates what can happen when congruence between the nurse and patient is lacking.

SCENARIO 3.1

Katie is 17 weeks pregnant and smokes 15 cigarettes per day. During a discussion with the nurse, Katie is able to articulate some of the reasons why she should give up smoking during pregnancy, indicating some health literacy about her behaviour. However, her nurse incorrectly identifies her as being in the contemplation phase, moving towards preparation, without checking and agreeing this with Katie. The nurse's conversation focuses on making a plan for behaviour change before fully exploring Katie's motivation to make this change. There is no congruence between patient and nurse and in turn, Katie shows resistance by becoming withdrawn and showing a lack of interest in the conversation.

When assessing motivation for change it is necessary to explore with your patient how important they feel this behaviour change is to them and how confident they feel to undertake the change. In the example in *Scenario 3.1*, Katie was indicating that she felt it was important to stop smoking but was not feeling confident to make this change at present. Her nurse needed to discuss how confident Katie was feeling about giving up smoking and what strategies would help her to improve her confidence and belief she could make this change.

Thinking carefully about our own skills in communicating with our patients at each step of the health promotion process, the OARS acronym in *Figure 3.2* is most effective in helping our patients to explore their motivation to change health behaviours.

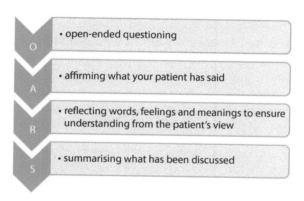

Figure 3.2 *The OARS acronym.*

These are the skills required to help move around the model of behaviour change and towards the planning and action stage and are discussed in depth in *Chapter 4*. Using open-ended questioning at the start of a conversation, such as 'How are you feeling about your health?' gives an individual choice to discuss a health issue or not, which in turn reveals what is important to your patient about their health choices. This style of listening will also help when a relapse has occurred. As already stated, relapse is an integral part of this behaviour change cycle and each time it occurs, the individual has an opportunity to reflect on why they relapsed. Discussing this with their nurse will help them to understand further the issues that caused them to relapse and enable a conversation about how to prevent this from happening next time they are trying to change their behaviour.

ACTIVITY 3.1

Consider a patient who is obese and is at risk of developing health complications because of this. How do you feel about instigating a conversation to assess the stage of motivation to change? Drawing on previous reading from this book, what styles of communication would be appropriate in this situation? What questions would you ask?

If the patient appears to be at the contemplation stage, how would you discuss and encourage the move to the next phase of planning for change? What resources are available in your area to support a plan of action?

You can also consider this model for your own health behaviours to consider a particular health issue. Which phase from the transtheoretical model do you think you are in?

How ready or motivated to change this behaviour are you? Remember to think about how important the change is to you and how confident you feel to make a change.

What would help you to move into the next phase of the model and how would you like this to be delivered?

3.3 Explaining an evidence-based approach to health

In order to explain an evidence-based approach to health to patients/clients, we first need to understand ourselves what this is and how it can best be employed within the role of the nurse. The NMC *Code* (Nursing and Midwifery Council, 2018) section 6 states: 'Always practise in line with the best available evidence'. To achieve this the nurse can:

- make sure any information or advice given is evidence-based, including information relating to using any healthcare products or services, and
- maintain the knowledge and skills you need for safe and effective practice.

An evidence-based approach to health can best be defined as: "the integration of the best research evidence with clinical expertise and the patient's preferences and values" (Sackett *et al.*, 2000).

This definition, although first published in 2000, remains relevant today. It suggests there are three components to evidence-based healthcare that can be viewed as a collaboration between research evidence, professional expertise, and patient values and understanding (*Figure 3.3*).

Our patients expect that all nurses understand the care they are delivering and are able to discuss and explain why this care or intervention is suitable for an individual. We need to be able to provide a thorough rationale about the care we are giving, based on the best available evidence, so a patient can be helped to make an

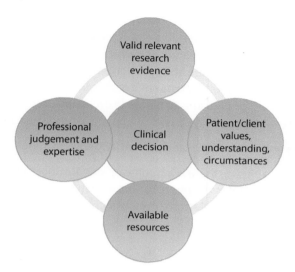

Figure 3.3 *The interdependence between the three key features described to aid decision-making.*

informed decision about their health. It is also necessary to base care on the most reliable and current evidence that is available, to ensure we remain 'accountable' for our practice. The NMC *Code* (Nursing and Midwifery Council, 2018) declares that 'nurses and midwives are accountable for the care that they deliver' so being able to justify your intervention based on the most relevant and current evidence will ensure that this element of the *Code* is adhered to.

As discussed above, Sackett *et al.* (2000) described how clinical decisions are also reliant on a professional's clinical judgement. This can be used to decide whether the best evidence can and should be applied to the individual patient/client, given each patient is an individual and in unique circumstances. Professional 'intuition' or 'gut feeling' was first described by Benner (1984) as being in a close relationship with experience. He claimed that intuition is grounded in both knowledge and experience and that in the absence of reliable research, professional judgement is the best available evidence on which to promote health and care. In a recent review conducted by Melin-Johansson *et al.* (2017), nursing intuition was found to be part of a process that is based on knowledge and experience and they suggested that it has a place alongside research-based evidence.

Finally, in Sackett's model, he describes the importance of listening to a patient/client's preferences, values and understanding about the care they could receive. Some clients wish to be fully involved in the decisions relating to the care they receive and for these patients, tools such as the NHS 111 website (https://111.nhs.uk) can be invaluable to support their understanding before or after we as nurses have discussed the care options. For all patients, it is vital that we gain their informed consent prior to an intervention or health promotion activity. Even with the most reliable research evidence available and discussed together with the nurse's professional judgement, if the patient/client chooses not to consent then this care/information cannot be given.

There are a few caveats to this, for example within the safeguarding arena of both children and vulnerable adults. Referral to statutory services for protection must take place to offer safety for the child or adult. It also applies where a patient has either temporarily or permanently lost the ability to consent, due to a learning disability, mental health illness, brain injury or dementia and the Mental Capacity Act (2005) is invoked. This Act allows for decisions to be made on behalf of such a patient by the providers of their care and is always based on the most current evidence available.

So how do nurses find valid reliable and current evidence to impart to their patients?

Within the field of healthcare, there is a significant debate about evidence and what type of study constitutes the best possible evidence of an intervention. Many authors use a pyramid to illustrate the hierarchy of evidence, as illustrated in *Figure 3.4*.

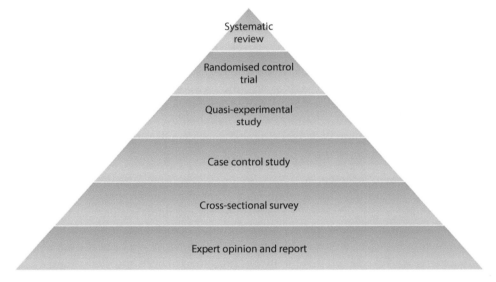

Figure 3.4 *The hierarchy of evidence.*

Within health and nursing research, systematic reviews are deemed to provide the gold standard of research. These are reviews of all the primary research available in a subject area, and the reviewers form a recommendation based on the findings from them all. The Cochrane Collaboration, which is a non-profit organisation with contributors worldwide, produces reviews that summarise the best available evidence generated through research to inform decisions about health. However, evidence-based programmes of health promotion tend to be of a quasi-experimental and cross-sectional study type where there is no comparison group of patients and the results are often interpreted with multiple caveats. Whichever evidence source we use, nurses need to be able to critically analyse the findings to decide whether the evidence is valid and reliable. There are many publications available that can help to support this analysis and nurses need to ensure they feel competent to undertake this with their patients.

Strategies for disseminating information are detailed in *Section 3.4*. However, it is important to consider how evidence-based practice is communicated verbally to patients in a clear, consistent way. You may have heard patients justifying a health activity or approach based on information gained from a friend or family member. They may also refer to a magazine or newspaper article they have read or web sources. It is important to acknowledge their understanding based on the information they have received and not dismiss this as trivial material. Building a trusting, respectful relationship will help to encourage dialogue about the types of evidence available and the trustworthiness of information relating to a patient's health needs. Some key points to consider in these situations are listed below. You may choose to use some or all of these, depending on the situation presented:

- Show an interest in the type of information drawn upon by the patient to help understand their viewpoint.
- Do not be dismissive of non-evidence-based information the patient believes to be true.
- Take time to explain the variety of information available and how robust research studies help to ensure a consensus of opinion based on the best possible evidence.
- Use clear, simple language that can be understood.
- Explain that you aim to provide the best care possible based on clinically researched evidence.
- Compare the information in a magazine to a clinically based research study to demonstrate differences.
- Discuss the history of ritual, tradition and personal choice in care and how this has progressed to evidence-based practice.
- Show how the advice or care you are giving relates to evidence-based practice.

ACTIVITY 3.2

Reflect on an episode of care where a patient needed to receive some information regarding a health-promoting activity. How was this undertaken? Was the information shared based on the most current evidence? How do you know this?

List four key points you would follow to ensure you impart current evidence-based healthcare.

3.4 Strategies for disseminating information (population and individual)

Since the rapid introduction of the internet and social media, the way health professionals, individuals and populations receive health information has changed radically. Prior to the proliferation of the worldwide web, most health staff received information from key health information sources such as government departments, research journals and the printed press. The information disseminated was one-directional and relied upon the professional sharing it with their patients/clients and local population in a timely manner (see *Figure 3.5*).

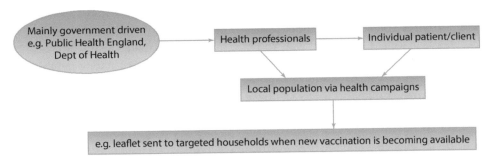

Figure 3.5 *Health information sources.*

This strategy of disseminating health information offered very little choice in the information shared to both an individual and at population level but was reliable and evidence-based. This was similarly seen by the adoption of mass media campaigns from the mid 1980s. These were often seen to present information in an alarmist way, an example being the 1986 'AIDS – Don't Die of Ignorance' TV campaign (www.youtube.com/watch?v=TMnb536WuC0). Again, the use of mass media as a strategy for sharing health information offered very little choice to the individual, although it was relatively successful in reaching the population as a whole.

We now need to find strategies that embrace the proliferation of new sources of information. Individuals can now obtain the information that they require from a wide range of sources and can also disseminate it to other interested parties, as described by Dumbrell and Steele (2013). This means that health information can be shared in a more dynamic manner and this is illustrated in *Figure 3.6*.

As social media is playing more of a role in informing and engaging our patients in their healthcare decision-making, nurses should question the reliability of the

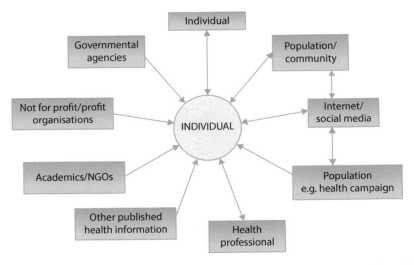

Figure 3.6 *The sharing of health information, offering choice to both individual and population.*

information that is being shared and whether individuals have the critical appraisal skills required to make sense of the vast amounts of information available.

A study of primary care nurses by Bekkum and Hilton (2013) found that media influence can have a detrimental effect on an individual's decision-making as there is not always sufficient unbiased information presented. Nurses need to use their knowledge to help their patients/clients to understand what the research behind the headlines is actually saying. One example is a recent cohort study by Sabia *et al.* (2018) which looked at alcohol consumption and the risk of a dementia diagnosis. The headline in the press and on various social media platforms was: "Middle-aged non-drinkers may have 'higher risk' of dementia", whereas the actual study published in the *British Medical Journal* was entitled "Alcohol consumption and risk of dementia: 23 year follow-up of Whitehall II cohort study".

In order to help a patient/client have a full understanding of this piece of research, the nurse needs to draw upon her critical appraisal skills and a range of communication strategies to ensure that the individual does not see this as a reason to start drinking alcohol, for example.

As we know that people are increasingly using social networks to exchange and search for health information, our strategy for promoting health needs to engage with this medium. Health organisations, professionals and academics can use these platforms to promote the correct information when mass media is covering an area in a more biased way. By regular dissemination of information regarding promoting healthy behaviours, a wide array of individuals and local populations can be reached.

Another strategy that could be employed to communicate reliable health information to the wider population is to use social media platforms in a more rapid and coordinated manner. Recently Twitter has become a popular source of health information (Hughes, 2016). Hughes suggested that recognised healthcare organisations such as Public Health England and academics can share current reliable information in a very timely manner, which would help our patients/clients to have more of the facts when the headlines hit!

However, we do need to be aware of the level of literacy required by the audience when sharing information in this form, and organisations and professionals sharing health information need to be clear in their profile that their information is evidence-based and of a robust nature, to help patients/clients/nurses identify the highest-quality information.

Health professionals such as nurses need to be aware of the varying quality of information available through Twitter and other social media platforms and be prepared to discuss this information with their patients, who may have accessed information and need help to interpret and understand what the information means for their own health decisions.

A further consideration of relying on social media for health information dissemination is that some groups of patients may not be able to access this technology. These groups may in fact be the target audience. The elderly and those with poor literacy skills or English as a second language may still need to be offered health promotion in a more traditional form as discussed earlier in this chapter, such as a face-to-face consultation with a health professional, with some information given in printed form and translated as required. This can enable them to make a more informed decision about their health at their own pace.

Younger members of the population are very quick to adopt the latest and differing social media platforms, compared to their parents and so only using one form of social media could exclude groups. Therefore organisations must offer multiple ways to disseminate and communicate key health promotion messages to be understood by both the individual and population concerned.

ACTIVITY 3.3

Make a list of the social media platforms you know and also ask colleagues. Now look at health-related posts and blogs within these platforms. How accessible is the platform to navigate and how did you appraise the quality of the information presented? How is the information communicated to the audience? Would you consider using any of these to help communicate or reinforce health messages with your patients?

What skills do you feel are required by the nurse to ensure patients can interpret, understand and make an informed decision regarding their healthcare?

3.5 Addressing common health risk behaviours

Life expectancy is rising within the UK. Men can now expect to live until 79.5 years of age and women to 83.1 years. That is the good news. Unfortunately, due to our health behaviours the population as a whole is spending more of this extra life unwell, with as much as 16 years of ill health for men and 19 years for women (Public Health England, 2019). What we are dying from is changing too. Whilst heart disease and stroke remain common causes of death, the number of patients dying with dementia and Alzheimer's disease has increased by 50–60%. We have an ageing population and this is putting a strain on all our health and social care services. Therefore we need to help our patients and clients to address their health risk behaviours and start making more healthy choices and adopting a healthier lifestyle.

The common health risk behaviours are well recognised and discussed frequently by the media, health professionals and governmental agencies. The key areas that contribute to the highest proportion of ill health are:

- consuming a diet high in calories, fat and sodium, and low in nutrients
- low levels of physical activity and high levels of sedentary behaviour
- smoking cigarettes
- abusing substances including alcohol, and prescription and illicit drugs

An individual and in turn the population could reduce these health behaviours. Statistics suggest that heart disease, stroke and type 2 diabetes could be prevented by up to 80% and cancers by 40%. The Global Burden of Disease report, based on findings from 1990 to 2016, highlighted the incidence of poor health and older age occurring within the various regions of the UK (Steel *et al.*, 2018). They provide some evidence to suggest that smoking in women is the number one risk factor for ill health for this half of the population and that poor diet coupled with smoking were the largest contributors to the number of deaths globally.

3.5.1 Making Every Contact Count (MECC)

One public health approach to trying to address these common health risk behaviours is Making Every Contact Count (MECC). This approach is supported by Public Health England (PHE) and Health Education England (HEE) and focuses on the lifestyle issues that can make the greatest positive change to an individual's health in a non-directive way.

> '*Making Every Contact Count (MECC) is an approach to behaviour change that uses the millions of day-to-day interactions that organisations and people have with other people to support them in making positive changes to their physical and mental health and wellbeing.*'

(Public Health England, NHS England and Health Education England, 2016)

MECC aligns well with many of PHE's priorities – stopping smoking, drinking alcohol within the recommended limits (14 units per week for men and women with some days of no alcohol each week), eating more healthily (reducing sugar, eating five or more portions of fruit and vegetables a day), being more physically active (10 minutes of brisk exercise per day), keeping to a healthy weight and improving mental health and wellbeing. It can also help with achieving the *Five Year Forward View* (NHS, 2014) principle of keeping the ageing population healthier and independent for longer.

Figure 3.7 is a diagrammatic representation of MECC and behaviour change interventions. It is envisaged that all health and social care staff will be trained and able to offer very brief and brief interventions to the patients and clients they see every day and that from signposting them on to more specialist professionals, we can start to make some difference to our nation's health.

What does a brief intervention look like?

A brief intervention, as discussed in *Chapter 2*, can happen anywhere and at any time. It aims to raise awareness, stimulate thinking and signpost to other information or agencies. Using the OARS acronym in a brief intervention could be the start of a patient thinking about making a move towards a healthier behaviour.

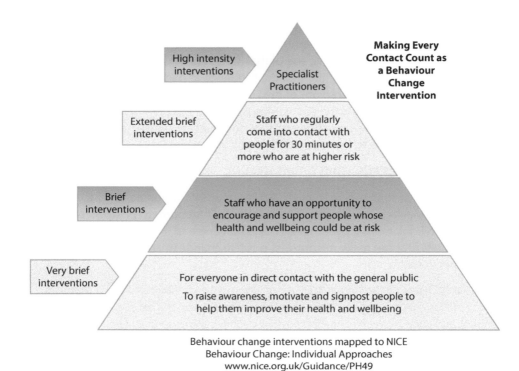

Behaviour change interventions mapped to NICE
Behaviour Change: Individual Approaches
www.nice.org.uk/Guidance/PH49

Figure 3.7 *Representation of Making Every Contact Count and behaviour change interventions.*

SCENARIO 3.2: A BRIEF INTERVENTION

A student nurse, James, is working within a GP practice nurse placement. He notices a patient who attended the diabetes clinic with the practice nurse and himself the week before. The patient is reading a leaflet on healthy eating.

James: open-ended question: Hello Mrs Jones. I see you've been looking at one of our leaflets about healthy eating. I remember we were discussing this with you last week. How have you been getting on with the diet sheet we gave you?

Patient: Not very well actually. It doesn't have any of the foods that I like and it's very confusing.

James: affirming and reflecting: Oh, I see. It sounds like you're not finding the information helpful and are looking for something that is more relevant to you.

Patient: Yes, that's right. I want something that helps me with foods that I like to eat.

James: Summarising and signposting: OK, shall we see what information we have here and whether any of it is more helpful? We could also look at the Change4Life and Diabetes UK websites for more information.

Patient: That would be great. I've been worrying about coming back to see the nurse today as I haven't been getting on at all well with it.

ACTIVITY 3.4

Can you think of a time in practice where you could have used the MECC approach to discuss a patient/client's health behaviour as a brief intervention?

If you were in a similar situation again, how might you start a conversation with the patient/client, and could you follow the OARS acronym to complete the brief intervention?

Make an aide memoire card with OARS written on it to keep in your pocket until this conversation becomes more familiar to you. You could have some agencies/information sources on the back for the most common health behaviours discussed earlier. Remember the more you practise this type of conversation, the easier it will become.

CASE STUDY

You and a family nurse are visiting a young client, who we will call Jody, as part of the Family Nurse Partnership programme (FNP, 2018). Jody commenced weaning of her baby at 11 weeks. The Department of Health guidelines (2018) state that exclusive breastfeeding until 6 months is best for baby. There is some evidence that has shown that the early introduction of solid food has long-term consequences for the health of that individual, with a higher incidence of gut allergies and obesity (World Health Organization, 2002). The Department of Health's guidelines are based on this WHO research.

Up until this stage Jody had exclusively breastfed her baby, but he had started waking at night and she had read in one of the daily newspapers that commencing solid food might help her baby to sleep better. She had also discussed the issue with her mum, who had reinforced this decision as she herself had introduced solids at around 3 months with each of her children. At a regular home visit at 12 weeks, Jody tells you and the nurse about the decision she has made and explained her reasons.

What would you and the nurse do in this instance? What initial conversations could be had and what approach could be taken?

What stage of the transtheoretical change model do you think Jody could be at this point? How could you ensure congruency with Jody to build a trusting relationship?

Thinking about what this meant for Jody, you and the nurse decide to ask Jody whether she would like to look at some reliable evidence around introducing solid food. Jody gives her consent so you are able to share the current weaning guidelines and further explore what Jody's baby might be telling her regarding the breastfeeding and sleeping. At around 3 months of age, her nurse knows from professional expertise and evidence that the baby is possibly in a growth period and may be asking for more frequent feeds to stimulate Jody's breast to increase the supply of milk to match this growth. This is discussed in the material produced by the Department of Health and so aids the nurse's sharing of this knowledge in a way acceptable to Jody. Using the technique of 'Elicit–Provide–Elicit' (described earlier in this chapter), Jody is able to understand the supply and demand feature of breastfeeding and accept that this is normal for her baby at this age.

CASE STUDY (*continued*)

At the end of this discussion, Jody informs you and the nurse that she thought her baby was not yet developmentally ready for solid food and that she was going to concentrate on her breastfeeding and wait until he showed signs of needing more before commencing weaning again. However, she felt pressured by family and friends as they had always done things that way with their babies.

What information would you leave with Jody to support her decision? Think about the types and format of information she would be able to access, such as websites, written articles, leaflets. Are they evidence-based? How would you explain the differences between an evidence-based approach and a custom and practice approach?

At the next visit two weeks later, Jody reported that she had stopped offering solid food to her baby and he had settled back into a more normal routine of feeding 2–3 hourly during the day and 3–4 hourly at night. The nurse felt that this was a positive reinforcement of Jody's healthcare decision and the fact that they were both much less tired and distressed, was a good evaluation of the discussion two weeks previously.

Jody did not introduce solid food to her baby's diet until he was 25 weeks old after reading the guidelines left by her nurse and using government social media platforms for information. She told her family and friends about this in order to share and justify her approach. Jody had also found information about baby-led weaning on the internet and wanted to discuss this with you and her nurse to understand whether this was reliable information and relevant for her and her baby.

This case study illustrates how important it is to assess an individual's motivation for change prior to offering health information, influencing factors which could affect decision-making such as family and friends in this instance, and then to use communication techniques to help understand the situation from the client's perspective. Using the most reliable and up to date evidence-based information, alongside professional expertise and client knowledge and understanding, allowed this mother to make an informed decision about the health of her baby. This in turn may reduce poor health outcomes for this child in later life and will ensure subsequent children that this mother has will be offered the same health decision regarding feeding.

Summary

This chapter has discussed some of the communication skills that a nurse might use to aid health promotion with their patients. It is important to remember that health values and beliefs are individual and as nurses, we must recognise that not everyone will want or believe they need to change unhealthy behaviours, despite overwhelming evidence. An honest, trusting relationship is fundamental to encourage a partnership approach in health promotion activities, but it is also important to realise that brief interventions can be as powerful as sustained health behaviour strategies.

KEY LEARNING POINTS

Four key points to take away from *Chapter 3*:

- ☑ Models of health promotion can help to structure health promotion activity with your patients, in particular the transtheoretical cycle of change.
- ☑ Always use the most current evidence base, but be mindful that new research is frequent.
- ☑ Communication of information must be adapted to the needs of the individual or group to ensure it is meaningful and understood.
- ☑ MECC can be a useful approach to draw on in any setting to focus on lifestyle issues.

FURTHER READING

Corcoran, N. (ed.) (2013) *Communicating Health: strategies for health promotion*, 2nd edition. Sage Publications.

Naidoo, J. and Wills, J. (2016) *Foundations of Health Promotion*, 4th edition. Elsevier Health Sciences.

Scrivens, A. (2017) *Ewles & Simnett's Promoting Health: a practical guide*, 7th edition. Elsevier Health Sciences.

REFERENCES

Bandura, A. (1977) Self-efficacy: toward a unifying theory of behavioral change. *Psychological Review*, **84(2)**: 191–215.

Bekkum, J.E. and Hilton, S. (2013) Primary care nurses' experiences of how the mass media influence frontline healthcare in the UK. *BMC Family Practice*, **14**: 178. Available at: https://doi.org/10.1186/1471-2296-14-178 (accessed 19 July 2019).

Benner, P. (1984) *From Novice to Expert: excellence and power in clinical nursing practice*. Addison-Wesley Publishing Company.

Department of Health (2018) *Your baby's first solid foods*. Available at: www.nhs.uk/conditions/pregnancy-and-baby/solid-foods-weaning (accessed 19 July 2019).

Dumbrell, D. and Steele, R. (2013) The changing nature of health information dissemination through the role of social media. *Applied Mechanics and Materials*, **411–14**: 110–14.

Family Nurse Partnership (2018) *A home visiting programme for first-time young mums and families*. Available at: https://fnp.nhs.uk (accessed 19 July 2019).

Hughes, E. (2016) Can Twitter improve your health? An analysis of alcohol consumption guidelines on Twitter. *Health Information Library Journal*, **33(1)**: 77–81.

Melin-Johansson, C., Palmqvist, R. and Rönnberg, L. (2017) Clinical intuition in the nursing process and decision-making – a mixed-studies review. *Journal of Clinical Nursing*, **26(23–24)**: 3936–49. Available at: https://doi.org/10.1111/jocn.13814

Miller, R.W. and Rollnick, S. (2012) *Motivational Interviewing: helping people change*, 3rd edition. The Guilford Press.

NHS (2014) *Five Year Forward View*. Available at: www.england.nhs.uk/wp-content/uploads/2014/10/5yfv-web.pdf (accessed 19 July 2019).

Nursing and Midwifery Council (2018) *The Code: professional standards of practice and behaviour for nurses, midwives and nursing associates*. NMC. Available at: www.nmc.org.uk/globalassets/sitedocuments/nmc-publications/nmc-code.pdf (accessed 19 July 2019).

Prochaska, J.O. and DiClemente, C.C. (1983) Stages and processes of self-change of smoking: toward an integrative model of change. *Journal of Consulting and Clinical Psychology*, 51: 390–5.

Public Health England (2019) *Health Matters: prevention, a life course approach*. Available at: www.gov.uk/government/publications/health-matters-life-course-approach-to-prevention (accessed 19 July 2019)

Public Health England, NHS England and Health Education England (2016) *Making Every Contact Count (MECC): consensus statement*. Available at: www.england.nhs.uk/wp-content/uploads/2016/04/making-every-contact-count.pdf (accessed 19 July 2019).

Sabia, S., Fayosse, A., Dumurgier, J. *et al.* (2018) Alcohol consumption and risk of dementia: 23 year follow-up of Whitehall II cohort study. *British Medical Journal*, **362**: k2927. doi: https://doi.org/10.1136/bmj.k2927

Sackett, D.L., Straus, S.E., Richardson, W.S., Rosenberg, W.M. and Haynes, R.B. (2000) *Evidence-Based Medicine: How to Practice and Teach EBM*. Churchill Livingstone.

Steel, N., Ford, J.A., Newton, J.N. *et al.* (2018) Changes in health in the countries of the UK and 150 English Local Authority areas 1990–2016: a systematic analysis for the Global Burden of Disease Study 2016. *Lancet*, **392**: 1647–61.

World Health Organization (1986) *The Ottawa Charter for Health Promotion*. First International Conference on Health Promotion, Ottawa, 21 November 1986.

World Health Organization (2002) *Fifty-fifth World Health Assembly. Infant and young child nutrition*. Available at: http://apps.who.int/gb/archive/pdf_files/WHA55/ewha5525.pdf (accessed 19 July 2019).

World Health Organization (2017) *The Mandate for Health Literacy*. Available at: www.who.int/healthpromotion/conferences/9gchp/health-literacy/en/ (accessed 19 July 2019).

Chapter 4

Communication skills for therapeutic intervention

Erica Pavord

LEARNING OUTCOMES

By the end of this chapter you should be able to:

4.1 Recognise the importance of therapeutic communication and identify ways in which to develop a therapeutic relationship

4.2 Understand key techniques used in motivational interviewing

4.3 Recognise key techniques used in reminiscence therapy

4.4 Explain effective de-escalation strategies and techniques

4.5 Appreciate how effective distraction and diversion strategies can be used.

4.1 Introduction

The communication and relationship management skills section of *Future Nurse: standards of proficiency for registered nurses* (Nursing and Midwifery Council, 2018, p. 29) requires nurses to use evidence-based, best practice communication skills and approaches for providing therapeutic interventions. Some of these skills are required within specialist settings and require specialist skills and knowledge. The approaches and techniques that are important in all adult healthcare settings are outlined in this chapter.

4.2 Developing a therapeutic relationship

As described in much of this book, communication in your career as a nurse will involve listening for information; assessing and evaluating; sharing information and advice. Therapeutic communication is different in that its purpose is simply to build trust and to connect with another person in a warm, accepting and genuine way. The word therapy, Greek in origin, means 'healing' and in this context it is concerned with healing of the mind rather than the body. This might explain why the word 'therapeutic' tends to be associated with counselling and psychotherapy. However, communicating therapeutically is a vital component of effective communication in nursing and many other health and social care settings.

Counselling and psychotherapy research and literature has focused much on the therapeutic relationship and how fundamental it is to the therapeutic encounter and to the outcomes of therapy. Regardless of modality, it is acknowledged that the relationship itself is the one common and essential component of successful outcomes (Charura and Paul, 2014). Given that in many health and social care settings much counselling takes place informally, away from the counselling room and within patient–practitioner relationships, it seems reasonable to assume that patient wellbeing and satisfaction will be linked to the quality of the relationships encountered whilst in the care of health practitioners.

Communicating therapeutically is as much about our *way of being* as it is about what we do or say. Carl Rogers, a key figure of the person-centred approach, entitled one of his seminal works 'A Way of Being' and in it wrote about communication at a 'feeling level' and of listening to another in such a way that we are able to hear the sounds and sense the shape of their inner world (Rogers, 1980, pp. 6–7). When we are with someone whose interactions with us are therapeutic in nature, we are more likely to feel a sense of safety and satisfaction. We feel listened to and understood at a level that enables us to feel validated and strengthened or we simply feel more able to go on with the challenges we face. This is a collaborative relationship with mutual understanding and trust at its core. The people in a relationship are partners, connected by a shared understanding of the issues and difficulties that are being discussed.

This description might sound like the therapeutic relationship is only achieved through some kind of elusive and innate quality in the practitioner, but it is not exclusive to counsellors and psychotherapists; it is expressed in many different ways through both verbal and non-verbal communication and can take place in any number of settings. It can be built through the use of active listening skills underpinned by sensitive, insightful reflective practice. At the roots of the therapeutic relationship are Rogers' three core conditions: empathy, unconditional positive regard or non-judgemental acceptance, and congruence, often referred to as genuineness (Rogers, 1957).

4.2.1 Empathy

Empathy is the ability to walk in another's shoes and to show a deep understanding of another's frame of reference. When we are empathetic we are able to follow and understand another person's subjective experience and respond to them without the filter of our own thoughts, feelings and experiences. Empathy is very different from sympathy, which too often is experienced as pity and can disempower us and leave us feeling helpless.

4.2.2 Unconditional positive regard

Unconditional positive regard is a way of being that is non-judgemental, warm and accepting of another person. People will inevitably withdraw and feel defensive if they sense they are being judged, so a therapeutic relationship cannot develop. In some circumstances it can feel difficult to avoid being judgemental when a person is communicating their distress through aggressive or rude or rejecting behaviour or through withdrawing and isolating themselves. In these situations, it can help to reflect on what feeling their behaviour might be communicating. If they feel afraid, sad, threatened or rejected it is understandable that they will want to keep people at a distance. It helps to be curious rather than judgemental about people. Genuine curiosity about what their behaviour might be communicating can help us to respond in an empathetic and accepting way.

4.2.3 Congruence

Congruence, genuineness or realness is a way of being that Rogers describes as a 'lifelong task' (1980, p. 14). If we can be fully ourselves and the person we are with experiences us as truly genuine it is more likely that he or she will be able to be genuine back. Being genuine is not easy; sometimes it is necessary for us to wear different 'hats' depending on where we are or who we are with, but genuineness is felt at a deeper level. We have all been in situations when the person we are communicating with is clearly trying hard to be something they are not, and in these situations it can be hard to trust them and to feel that they are with us. When we are genuine, we are able to communicate with another without a façade.

ACTIVITY 4.1

Think about a time when you have been a patient in a healthcare setting or know someone who has received care or treatment. This could be in a hospital setting, in the home, at a GP surgery, with a school nurse, or in a clinic setting. How did you feel about the situation? What do you think was needed from the healthcare professionals?

Now think about how they communicated that. What worked and didn't work so well?

It is likely that you felt concerned, worried, fearful or possibly bored. You might have felt relieved if you had waited a long time for this appointment; it's possible that you felt quite lonely and lacking in confidence. You might have felt that you were somehow in the way or taking up someone's time. In reflecting on what you felt you would need it's possible that you would want to feel listened to and respected and secure in the knowledge that the experts were taking care of you. Collins (2009, p. 11) suggested that through effective and therapeutic communication a patient can:

- be reassured
- feel that they are taken seriously
- feel able to understand their illness more fully
- voice their concerns
- feel empowered
- be motivated to follow up a medication regime
- express a desire to have treatment (or not)
- be given time and treated with respect.

It is hard to imagine that someone could feel this way in a relationship that is motivated simply by the desire and need to communicate essential information and advice in the most concise and efficient way. It is only possible to give people this experience through a warm, accepting and genuine therapeutic relationship. The interventions and techniques described in the rest of this chapter are only likely to be effective if a positive therapeutic relationship has been built between practitioner and patient.

4.3 **Motivational interviewing**

Rogers' core conditions are at the root of the motivational interviewing approach, which was developed by William R. Miller and Stephen Rollnick in the 1980s and designed to strengthen a person's motivation to bring about change in their lives. Motivational interviewing (MI) is an evidence-based, person-centred counselling style initially used in the field of substance misuse but now successfully used in numerous health and social care settings with people who are ambivalent about change.

It is safe to assume that the majority of people have aspects of their lifestyles that they know could be improved upon. We might say to ourselves things like: 'I need to eat less sugar' or 'I need to start exercising more regularly'. We all know what we should be doing more or less of so why don't we make the changes necessary? Perhaps it is because we are ambivalent about change. Miller and Rollnick (2012, p. 6) tell us that "ambivalence is simultaneously wanting and not wanting something, or wanting both of two incompatible things". When supporting people to make important changes in their lives we need to recognise that they are likely to know very well the things that they should be changing, so explaining why they have to make the changes and telling them how to do it is usually pointless because we are simply reiterating what they have already told themselves many times.

'You have to give up smoking. It's really bad for you and your family. You just need to be strong.' It is hard to imagine that there are many people who continue to smoke because they don't realise it's not good for them. It is more likely they continue to smoke because they are ambivalent about the huge change it would involve.

ACTIVITY 4.2

Think of a health or lifestyle change that you want to make. Make a list of the reasons why you want to change this aspect of your life. Then make a list of the reasons why this change has been difficult to make. As you read through this section reflect on the things that other people have said that have kept you stuck in ambivalence. Then reflect on the things that people have said that have helped you to make changes. Compare the things the more helpful people have said with the techniques outlined in this section.

The MI approach, like the person-centred approach, holds a fundamental assumption that we have inside us the strength to change our lives; it also argues that it is how we draw out the strength and motivation to change that makes a difference and improves outcomes. There are four key processes in MI that are needed to support patients to make necessary changes in their lives, as shown in *Figure 4.1*.

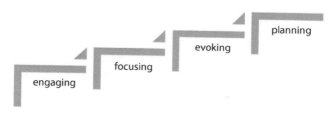

Figure 4.1 *Illustration of the central and overlapping processes that form the flow of MI.*

Miller and Rollnick (2012) describe these processes as both sequential and recursive; each step builds on those that were laid down before and continue to run beneath the process as it progresses. In the course of a conversation we might move up and down the steps as needed.

4.3.1 Engaging

In order to develop therapeutic relationships with people and to engage them in meaningful dialogue about their lives and the changes they want to make, we have to demonstrate our acceptance of them and our willingness to listen to what they tell us. Through warm, engaging and natural conversation, using active listening skills we begin a dialogue about that person's life and feelings about the difficulties they face.

4.3.2 Focusing

When people feel that we are with them and have a belief in them, they are more able to focus on a particular agenda. Focusing is the process by which you develop and maintain a specific direction in the conversation about change (Miller and Rollnick, 2012, p. 27). Through focusing people identify one or more change goals; these may involve behaviour changes or sometimes changes of attitude or choice.

4.3.3 Evoking

This step is at the heart of MI and involves an exploration of people's own motivations for change. Through thoughtful questioning you will focus on a particular goal and they will explore their own ideas and feelings about why and how they might bring about change. In some situations patients actively want our advice on the best action to take and are happy to take it but often there is resistance to change. Evoking is encouraging the patient to share their own reasons and arguments for change so that they talk *themselves* into it.

4.3.4 Planning

Throughout the process of focusing and evoking motivation for change people inevitably start to think about what action they will take to make the change happen. Through exploration and discussion they will begin thinking about what they might do and what it will be like when they have made changes. Planning involves commitment to change and formulating a plan of action that comes from their own ideas. The collaborative process elicits the person's own solutions and develops their autonomy.

Miller and Rollnick (2012) tell us that in conversation with people we will find ourselves moving in and out of the four processes of engaging, focusing, evoking and planning, sometimes within one conversation. Cutting across the four processes described above are the core skills that are particularly important in the person-centred approach. In MI these skills are known as OARS:

- **O**pen questions
- **A**ffirming
- **R**eflecting
- **S**ummarising

4.3.5 Open questions

Open questions help you to facilitate therapeutic communication through exploring ideas, thoughts and feelings. If someone asks 'Do you want to lose weight?' your answer can be either yes, no or I don't know. A question like that can feel challenging and judgemental and if we tend to be compliant with health professionals, we are likely to just say yes because that is what they want us to say. If the same person asks you 'What would it be like to lose weight?' you are encouraged to reflect on the possible advantages and disadvantages of losing weight. Questions like this are key in evoking motivation and beginning to plan change.

4.3.6 Affirming

Carl Rogers (1961, p. 17), in writing about the importance of acceptance, tells us: "The curious paradox is that when I accept myself just as I am, then I can change." It is difficult to make changes when we feel bad about ourselves, when we feel criticised and judged. It is a natural reaction to defend ourselves in the face of negativity and so we might withdraw, avoid or get angry. Through therapeutic communication, acceptance and affirmation we can help people to feel ready to accept themselves and to start to make changes.

The MI approach recognises that we all have strengths and resources and it is these that will facilitate and motivate change. Rather than judge or criticise we need to show a genuine respect for someone's abilities and good intentions. Through affirming comments, we bolster their effort and determination: 'I think it's so impressive that you have stuck to this eating plan for a whole week.' We can also make affirming statements through positive reframing. If a man tells you that he had a cigarette the day before after three days of no smoking, rather than say; 'Oh that's a shame, how disappointing'; you might say 'How did you manage to have just one cigarette in four days? That must have taken some willpower.' Through this reframing technique he hears his words reflected back to him in a positive, affirming way.

4.3.7 Reflecting

Throughout this book the importance of listening to people will have been repeated many times. Reflecting is a way of demonstrating our acceptance and empathy in such a way that the person we are listening to feels truly heard and understood. When we use reflection well, we are able to foster thoughtful exploration. Someone might be telling us about going for the first walk after returning home from having heart surgery.

Them: I really worried about going out, I could shuffle around at home but hadn't been outside for over two weeks. I nearly talked myself out of it and I got angry with my wife for pushing me.

You: It felt quite scary to go outside after your surgery.

Them: Yes, I was scared but didn't want to admit it.

You: You want people to think you are OK.

Them: Yes, I don't like feeling weak.

You: It's hard to show weakness when you are used to being strong.

Them: Yes, silly really, everyone knows what I've been through, I should probably ask for help.

Notice how the simple reflections help him to explore his feelings in a gentle and accepting way and lead him to thinking about doing something differently.

4.3.8 Summarising

Summarising is a bit like a long reflection. It is way of demonstrating that you have heard someone and got a sense of what they have been saying. It allows them to organise their thoughts and to make links to other ideas they have discussed. It can be a way of allowing them to hear and reflect on aspects of their experiences and to gain alternative perspectives and ideas. It can really illustrate the ambivalence people can have about change. A summary like this might be given at the end of a conversation with a patient who has to change their diet after a diagnosis of type 2 diabetes:

So, we've been talking about the impact of your recent diagnosis. It sounds like whilst it was a big shock to you, you are aware that your weight has been an issue for quite a long time. You know exactly what you need to do to change your diet because you have friends and family who have been through it and have managed to lose weight and keep it off. You know they will support you so you don't understand why it has been so hard to take the plunge. You feel really low sometimes and this has affected your self-esteem. Making important changes feels really huge and difficult and you aren't sure if you are up for it yet. Do you think I've got that right?

In offering a summary like this a person is able to stand back and gain a perspective on their difficulties that might be hard to do when they are in the middle of them. They are able to reflect on their 'stuckness' and explore potential new directions.

MI techniques like thoughtful questioning and reflecting skills from someone experienced can look like completely natural communication but it is skilled work and needs practice, plenty of careful listening and open and honest self-reflection.

4.4 Reminiscence therapies

Erik Erikson's (1950) theory of psychosocial development suggested that the final of his psychosocial stages involves a negotiation between either 'ego integrity' or 'despair'. This stage begins at age 65 and continues until death. During this period our lives slow down and we spend time contemplating our experiences and relationships. If through this process of contemplation and reflection we feel a sense of satisfaction and accomplishment we are more likely to experience ego integrity and accept our 'life cycle as something that had to be' (Erikson, 1950, p. 268). If on the other hand we look back at our lives and feel that we were unproductive or if we feel guilty about past events, we are likely to develop a sense of despair that can lead to loneliness and depression.

Most of us feel a sense of both ego integrity and despair; we alternate between the two, accepting our lives for what they are. Erikson's theory helps us to understand why reminiscence therapy techniques, used carefully, are a useful way to support people in the later stages of their lives.

Reminiscence therapy has its roots in the work of Butler's early work on life review (1963), which he describes as a process by which someone looks back on their life and reflects on past experiences. This person-centred process is particularly helpful for older people "in promoting a sense of integrity and adjustment" (Woods et al., 2018, p. 2). Zhou et al. (2011, p. 441) describe it as "using the recall of past events, feelings and thoughts to facilitate pleasure, quality of life or adaptation to present circumstances".

In the 1980s reminiscence work was introduced to dementia care and involves the use of familiar items from the past, such as photographs, household items, music and archive sound recordings to enhance interaction and generate discussion. It is usually carried out in a group, thereby encouraging people to share their memories and stories in an engaging and enjoyable way. The aim of reminiscence work is to create opportunities for interaction amongst people, between staff and patients, and between patients and others. These interactions aim to be meaningful, stimulating and enjoyable.

Reminiscence therapy is a popular intervention in dementia care, where it has been found to improve cognition, mood and wellbeing of those with mild to moderate dementia (Woods et al., 2018). There is also evidence that reminiscence work with family caregivers has helped to improve relationships and decrease caregiver stress (Woods et al., 2018). The benefits are not exclusive to dementia patients; Chiang et al. (2010) found that reminiscence therapy can lead to improvements in depression and loneliness and promote psychological wellbeing in older people without dementia.

4.4.1 Reminiscence therapy principles

In order for reminiscence work to be successful it must be underpinned by the following (Sim, 2003, p. 44):
- Effective communication and listening skills
- A commitment to spending time with people
- Having something interesting and meaningful to talk about

- Helping people with communication difficulties to communicate
- Being able to respond naturally and spontaneously in a positive way
- A holistic approach practised by a variety of staff, including management
- Time to prepare and review.

4.4.2 Reminiscence therapy resources

Resources must be appropriate to age, culture and background and within people's experience (*Table 4.1*).

Table 4.1 *The types of resources used in reminiscence work (adapted from Sim, 2003)*

Resource	Ways of using the resource
Photographs	These need to be clear and chosen purposefully, not just because they are old; they need to have relevance to the patients. Draw attention to aspects of the picture that will elicit discussion. You are looking for triggers that may evoke recognition, association, comparison, opinion and comment. The image might be used to initiate discussion about direct experience, e.g. a photograph of a high street in the patient's home town taken when they were a young person. You could ask them about the shops and buildings that were there, you could talk about the kinds of shops they liked to go to, how much things cost, how they got to the shops and how often.
Objects and memorabilia	It is a good idea to collect items that might elicit discussion about everyday life, about the locality, national and local events and personalities – old kitchen or garden implements, crockery, ornaments, books, items of clothing or old toys. Remember that the smell and texture of an object can evoke memories as much as its appearance. If you know your patients well you will have gathered information about their lives and their interests so you can be on the lookout for relevant memorabilia.
Audio or visual recordings and films	Start to collect recordings of social/historical programmes, which are often full of nostalgic and biographical excerpts. After watching a programme discuss what you have seen – you can stop and start it at appropriate parts to stimulate discussion about the content. If you have the right equipment you can get hold of old reel film, which immediately communicates the atmosphere of a particular era. Popular films with well-known film stars can bring collective memory together. Music from different eras is incredibly evocative and singing along or possibly dancing can bring people together in shared remembrance.

As with all therapeutic work the core conditions of empathy, acceptance and genuineness are at the foundation of reminiscence therapy. These conditions, demonstrated through active listening skills, are a key part of developing a warm rapport and communicating to patients their intrinsic value and worth as a person. The following is a reminder of those skills, with examples of how they might be used in the context of reminiscence work.

Be aware of non-verbal signals: if someone smiles or frowns or laughs in response to a reminiscence you need to notice it and reflect what you see: "I notice you're smiling as you look at that, I'm wondering what you are thinking about." People might signal that they are uncomfortable by turning away or crossing their arms; you need to be respectful of this.

Reflection and summary: Show that you have listened to the person by reflecting key aspects of the content and acknowledging any feelings that arise. Try to bring up information that you have heard in previous conversations to make links to what they are saying: "So, when you were just five years old you used to walk to your grandparents' house every Saturday, a five-mile round trip. That's a long way for a little boy! I remember you saying how close you were to them."

Use of questions: Remember that open questions invite more exploration than closed questions. Think of questions that begin with:

What: What was it like when you finished school?

How: How did you meet your husband?

Where: Where did you and your friends go to play when you were allowed out?

When people get upset

It can be concerning when someone's painful or upsetting memories are evoked through reminiscence activities. If this happens it is important to remember the core conditions of empathy, acceptance and genuineness and to use active listening skills as people talk about their difficult memories. It can be upsetting if someone has started to cry as a result of the activity but remember that crying is usually an appropriate and honest expression of the sadness and nostalgia they may feel. In these situations you need to be sensitive to non-verbal signals and respect someone's reluctance to continue. It is important not to make a fuss but to offer warm and empathetic reflection of their feelings. You could ask them if they want to go to a quieter place to talk with you; stay with them and give them the space to feel sad and to talk if they want to: "Reminiscence, by bringing to our consciousness people, places and moments that, except in our hearts, are gone forever, is likely to touch some tender places" (Sim, 2003, p. 59).

ACTIVITY 4.3

The next time you are working with an older person or maybe when you are talking to an older family member, choose an object or photograph and use some of the skills outlined in this chapter to initiate conversation. Focus your time on listening and asking open questions that are relevant to the discussion you have initiated.

Reflect on this activity: what feelings did it evoke in you? How engaged did you feel and how engaged do you think the elderly person felt? How could you tell?

4.5 De-escalation strategies and techniques

In any setting conflict is bound to arise at times when feelings are strong and there are differences in attitudes, values or needs. Conflict tends to involve two elements: the conflict issue and the emotional response to the situation (Arnold and Boggs,

2016). Lack of communication or poor communication is usually at the root of conflict and it is the responsibility of the professional to look for resolution.

Arnold and Boggs (2016, p. 244) suggest that there are five distinct styles of response to conflict:

Avoidance: Sometimes when a situation is uncomfortable or potentially threatening the most natural thing to do is to withdraw. Sometimes it might be appropriate to walk away if there is unlikely to be a satisfactory outcome from engaging with the conflict but there are times when this just postpones the inevitable.

Accommodation: We might want to avoid conflict at all costs and so we give in to another's demands by compromising our own needs or by giving false assurances. This might defuse the situation in the moment but rarely does it deal with the issue.

Competition: Some of us don't like to back down and feel like we must have the last word. In response to conflict we use our authority to suppress the conflict but this can lead to increased stress and further conflict.

Compromise: By compromising, each party in the conflict gives a little and takes a little. However, this is only effective when both parties hold equal power and this is often not the case when a patient is feeling vulnerable and dependent.

Collaboration: This is when we work together to find a mutually agreeable solution. It involves directly confronting the issue, acknowledging feelings and using open communication. We begin by identifying the concerns of each party, we work to clarify assumptions held by each person through honest communication, then we work collaboratively to find a solution that satisfies everyone.

The very nature of healthcare settings means that the people we support are likely to be experiencing feelings of fear, worry, anger, despair, sadness and exhaustion. Sometimes, in more positive situations, they might be experiencing huge feelings of relief or in neutral situations simply feelings of boredom. It is also important to remember that different cultures may regulate the display of emotion differently and so we might assume that someone is feeling something based on our own cultural expectations. It is these feelings and the way that we respond to them that can lead to conflict in healthcare settings.

Understanding the feeling that underlies someone's aggressive, angry response to us will help us to respond in a calm way, de-escalating the situation and creating an environment where the person feels heard and understood. Often the emotion we see, for example anger shown through shouting, masks a feeling of worry or even panic. Sometimes there is a mismatch between the emotion that we might see someone displaying and the feeling they are experiencing inside and so we respond to them inappropriately.

It is not only the feelings of others that are important in understanding how and why a situation escalates; it is also vital that we are aware of our own feeling states and are able to identify when a particular feeling is triggered in us and how we might respond to that trigger in a professional way. When we are in the presence of someone who is displaying emotions such as panic, anger or despair it can be stressful and sometimes frightening. If we respond to them in angry or frightened or dismissive ways, not only are we failing to communicate effectively, we are also behaving unprofessionally. However, it is very difficult to contain our own feelings of fear and anger when we are with someone who is abusing us either verbally or physically or who is threatening to harm themselves or others.

Pavord and Donnelly (2015, p. 107) offer the following guidelines when emotion is high and we are feeling threatened by someone's aggressive behaviour.

4.5.1 Verbal de-escalation

- Use a one-to-one approach
- Use the individual's name
- Ask open questions
- Enquire about the reason for the anger
- Don't be defensive even when abuse is directed at you
- Ask questions about facts rather than feelings
- Answer informational questions but avoid abusive ones
- Show concern and empathy, use active listening skills
- Acknowledge their grievances, concerns and frustrations but don't interpret or analyse their feelings
- Use slow clear speech
- Keep your volume and tone quiet and calm
- Don't patronise them, be respectful
- Give choices where appropriate.

4.5.2 Non-verbal de-escalation

- Maintain limited eye contact and a neutral facial expression
- Have open body language and minimise the gestures you use
- Allow greater body space than normal
- Consider the position of your body, be at the same eye level as the person, face them and ensure that you have clear access to the exit
- Minimise your movement, stay as still as possible
- Appear calm, self-controlled and confident without being dismissive or overbearing.

4.6 Distraction and diversion strategies

There will be times when you are supporting people who feel very anxious about procedures and who manage this through avoidance or through getting agitated or angry. It is useful to understand what they are experiencing and how to help them to manage this anxiety. When we feel threatened the 'fight or flight' mechanism is activated and it is more difficult to use rational thinking strategies. We sense danger and immediately our bodies prepare us for this danger. Some signs of this might be:

- Rapid heartbeat
- Sweating
- Tense muscles
- Stomach pain
- Quick, shallow breathing.

ACTIVITY 4.5

Reflect on a time when you have gone into fight or flight mode.

What physical symptoms did you notice? What did you do? What helps or hinders your recovery when you are in this state?

When people are in fight or flight mode we can help them to manage this with a number of distraction and diversion techniques; this gives their bodies time to return to a pre-arousal level and for their thinking to become more rational. Distraction and diversion techniques can support the patient to shift their attention

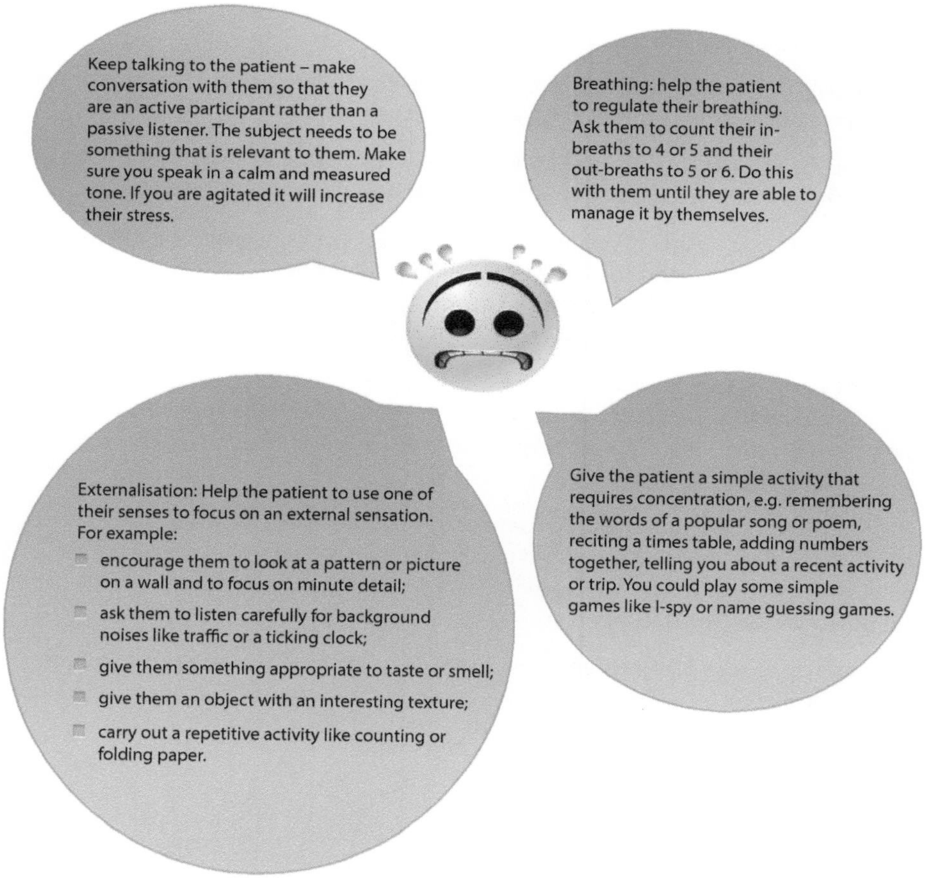

Keep talking to the patient – make conversation with them so that they are an active participant rather than a passive listener. The subject needs to be something that is relevant to them. Make sure you speak in a calm and measured tone. If you are agitated it will increase their stress.

Breathing: help the patient to regulate their breathing. Ask them to count their in-breaths to 4 or 5 and their out-breaths to 5 or 6. Do this with them until they are able to manage it by themselves.

Externalisation: Help the patient to use one of their senses to focus on an external sensation. For example:

- encourage them to look at a pattern or picture on a wall and to focus on minute detail;
- ask them to listen carefully for background noises like traffic or a ticking clock;
- give them something appropriate to taste or smell;
- give them an object with an interesting texture;
- carry out a repetitive activity like counting or folding paper.

Give the patient a simple activity that requires concentration, e.g. remembering the words of a popular song or poem, reciting a times table, adding numbers together, telling you about a recent activity or trip. You could play some simple games like I-spy or name guessing games.

Figure 4.2 *Examples of diversion and distraction techniques.*

away from the fear and towards something neutral or positive. *Figure 4.2* illustrates some of the techniques that can help patients to regulate their feelings of worry or panic and redirect their thoughts away from negativity and fear.

CASE STUDY

You are a student nurse whose final placement is a vascular outpatients unit.

Sally is a 58-year-old woman who attends the unit two afternoons a week for dressings to venous leg ulcers. She has osteoarthritis and has a body mass index of 33.

Sally lives alone and in the last two years has lost both her mother and father to cancer. She works as a primary school teacher and has been in the same school since she qualified 30 years ago. Due to Sally's pain and increasingly limited mobility, she has not been able to work for 3 months and is unsure when she will be able to return. She fears she might not be able to return at all. She clearly loves her job and speaks fondly about her colleagues and children at the school. She admits that her job is her life and has very little social life outside of this. She appears to be quite strong and positive about her diagnosis and always arrives well prepared for her appointment with books and crossword puzzles in case of delays. However, you have recently noticed that Sally seems quite distant when you talk to her and is spending less time reading and more time sitting silently, seemingly lost in her thoughts.

What feelings do you think Sally is experiencing at this time? How might you begin to develop a therapeutic relationship with Sally and how might it help her?

What aspects of Sally's life experience are likely to evoke difficult or upsetting feelings in you? How might you manage these while you develop a therapeutic relationship with her?

Six weeks into her treatment, you notice that Sally speaks more negatively about her life. She says that coming to the hospital/clinic is the highlight of her week – she laughs as she says it but then begins to cry. She cries for a short time but then grows angry and starts to tear up her crossword book, crumpling up the pages and throwing them across the room.

What do you think Sally is experiencing right now? What emotions is she showing and what might her feelings be? How might you respond to Sally when she first gets upset? What active listening skills will you use and why? What de-escalation techniques will you use to support Sally?

In a team meeting you share your concerns about Sally and the team discuss the possibility that she could be supported to take up activities that would enable her to meet people and socialise. Your supervisor asks you to research and discuss possible activities that Sally could take part in.

Look back at the key processes of engaging, focusing, evoking and planning and reflect on how you might help Sally to make changes in her life as she adjusts to her illness and manage its impact on her daily living.

Summary

A therapeutic relationship must be at the foundation of effective, patient-centred communication in healthcare settings and must ensure that patients feel listened to, understood and supported. Therapeutic relationships are underpinned by the core conditions of empathy, non-judgemental acceptance and genuineness. There are certain therapeutic techniques that are particularly important in most healthcare settings. MI techniques facilitate in patients a readiness and willingness to make important changes in their lives. Reminiscence therapy techniques support older patients to engage in enjoyable social interactions with those around them. Sometimes when conflict arises, emotions such as anger and panic can get in the way of effective communication and certain strategies are needed to defuse and distract from tension.

KEY LEARNING POINTS

Six key points to take away from *Chapter 4*:

- ☑ A supportive therapeutic relationship is a key component of positive outcomes for patients in healthcare settings.
- ☑ Use of person-centred active listening skills underpins the development of therapeutic relationships.
- ☑ MI techniques enable you to support patients to make necessary changes in their lives.
- ☑ Reminiscence therapy techniques use recall of past events to help to improve quality of life and relationships in older patients.
- ☑ De-escalation strategies help you to defuse conflict and manage your own feelings when patients are angry or very anxious.
- ☑ Distraction or diversion techniques help patients regulate overwhelming feelings when they are undergoing certain procedures.

FURTHER READING

Dart, M.A. (2011) *Motivational Interviewing in Nursing Practice: empowering the patient.* Jones & Bartlett Learning.

Gibson, F. (2011) *Reminiscence and Life Story Work: a practice guide*, 4th edition. Jessica Kingsley Publishers.

McCormack, B. and McCance, T. (2016) *Person-Centred Practice in Nursing and Health Care*, 2nd edition. John Wiley & Sons Ltd.

REFERENCES

Arnold, E. and Boggs, K.U. (2016) *Interpersonal Relationships: professional communication skills for nurses*, 7th edition. Elsevier.

Butler, R.N. (1963) The life review: an interpretation of reminiscence in the aged. *Psychiatry*, **26**: 65–76.

Charura, D. and Paul, S. (2014) *The Therapeutic Relationship Handbook: theory and practice*. McGraw-Hill Education.

Chiang, K.J., Chu, H., Chang, H.-J. *et al.* (2010) The effects of reminiscence therapy on psychological well-being, depression and loneliness among the institutionalized aged. *International Journal of Geriatric Psychiatry*, **25(4)**: 380–8.

Collins, S. (2009) Good communication helps to build a therapeutic relationship. *Nursing Times*, **105(24)**: 11.

Erikson, E. (1950) *Childhood and Society*. Norton.

Miller, W.R. and Rollnick, S. (2012) *Motivational Interviewing: helping people change*, 3rd edition. The Guilford Press.

Nursing and Midwifery Council (2018) *Future Nurse: standards of proficiency for registered nurses*. NMC. Available at: www.nmc.org.uk/globalassets/ sitedocuments/education-standards/future-nurse-proficiencies.pdf (accessed 19 July 2019).

Pavord, E. and Donnelly, E. (2015) *Communication and Interpersonal Skills*, 2nd edition. Lantern Publishing Ltd.

Rogers, C. (1957) The necessary and sufficient conditions for therapeutic change. *Journal of Consulting Psychology*, **21**: 95–103.

Rogers, C. (1961) *On Becoming a Person*. Houghton Mifflin.

Rogers, C. (1980) *A Way of Being*. Houghton Mifflin.

Sim, R. (2003) *Reminiscence: social and creative activities with older people in care*. Speechmark.

Woods, B., O'Philbin, L., Farrell, E.M., Spector, A.E. and Orrell, M. (2018) Reminiscence therapy for dementia. The Cochrane Database of Systematic Reviews, vol. 3, pp. CD001120.

Zhou, W., He, G., Gao, J. *et al.* (2011) The effects of group reminiscence therapy on depression, self-esteem and affect balance of Chinese community dwelling elderly. *Archives of Gerontology*, **54(3)**: 440–7.

Chapter 5

Communication skills in difficult situations

Louise Carter

LEARNING OUTCOMES

By the end of this chapter you should be able to:

5.1 Understand what is meant by the term communication vulnerable

5.2 Identify the intrinsic factors that can lead to a person being communication vulnerable

5.3 Recognise the extrinsic factors within the healthcare environment that may negatively impact on the communication vulnerable individual

5.4 Describe a range of nursing strategies that can be used to enhance communication with patients who have special communication needs.

5.1 Introduction

Where people have special communication needs or a disability, it is essential that reasonable adjustments are made in order to communicate, provide and share information in a manner that promotes optimum understanding and engagement and facilitates equal access to high quality care.

(NMC, 2018a, p. 18)

Most of us take the art of communication for granted. An essential aspect of life, we view it as a natural process that is central to a person's identity, self-esteem, social interactions and quality of life. Communication facilitates healthy social relationships, which in turn helps us maintain mental and physical health. Effective communication between nurse and patient is essential to person-centred and therapeutic care, ensuring that patients are active participants in their care, and can make informed choices.

Breakdown in communication can occur at any time along the healthcare continuum, in any setting, and can have an impact on not only the patient, but also the family, carers and health professional themselves.

This chapter will explore the concept of communication vulnerability and the factors that may affect communication across a range of caring scenarios. It will identify strategies that can be employed to help the nurse address these challenges in practice.

5.2 Demonstrating compassion and sensitivity

As a nurse, the development and maintenance of caring, compassionate and therapeutic relationships is the cornerstone to the provision of individualised, person-centred care. It is essential to the holistic assessment and understanding of your patients' needs, and to the overall quality of the care provided. The term therapeutic relationship is often referred to, but how do we define it? What do we mean by the therapeutic relationship, and why is it important to nursing? Dart (2011, p. 16) defines a therapeutic relationship as "one in which the patient feels comfortable being open and honest with the nurse".

Price (2017) identifies rapport and trust as the key components to the development of a therapeutic relationship. Rapport is described as the ability to establish and maintain a relationship, and this in turn leads to developing trust. In practice, this rapport and building of trust involves not only the patient, but also their family or carers. Therefore, the therapeutic relationship will involve a number of individuals and is dependent on skilful and sensitive communication.

The NMC *Code* (2018) presents the professional standards that nurses and midwives must uphold in order to be registered to practise in the UK. The *Code* requires nurses to ensure that "patient and public safety is protected", with Standard 17 stating that nurses have a duty to "raise concerns immediately if they believe a person is vulnerable or at risk and needs extra support and protection". To achieve this, nurses must (NMC, 2018):

- Take all reasonable steps to protect people who are vulnerable or at risk of harm, neglect, or abuse
- Share information if you believe someone may be at risk of harm, in line with the laws relating to the disclosure of information
- Have knowledge of and keep to the relevant laws and policies about protecting and caring for vulnerable people.

Therefore, nurses have a duty of care to ensure the needs of the vulnerable adult are safeguarded. So, let us consider what we mean by the term vulnerable adult. A vulnerable adult has been defined as:

> *Someone aged 18 or over: who is, or may be, in need of community services due to age, illness or a mental or physical disability. Who is, or may be, unable to take care of himself/herself, or unable to protect himself/herself against significant harm or exploitation.*

(Department of Health, 2015)

It is recognised that within healthcare provision vulnerable individuals may find it difficult to communicate their own decisions, and may require support to make fully informed choices about their own lives (Green, 2015; Stans *et al.*, 2013). As a result, we can define 'communication vulnerability' as a reduction in the capacity of an individual to hear, speak, see, read, write, understand or remember. This may be related to factors that are intrinsic to the individual, for example disabilities related to visual or hearing impairment; cognitive, receptive and expressive language skills. However, it may also be due to extrinsic factors, for example the environment or situation, that may also inhibit communication. *Table 5.1* identifies some of these intrinsic and extrinsic factors.

Table 5.1 *Factors that may lead to communication vulnerability*

Intrinsic	Extrinsic
Hearing impairment	Physical environment (noise, acoustics)
Visual impairment	Physical environment (lighting)
Dementia	Written information
Cerebral vascular accident (CVA)	Culture
Cancer of head and neck	Language
Traumatic brain injury	Perceptions of healthcare professionals
Progressive neurological conditions, e.g. Parkinson's disease, multiple sclerosis, motor neurone disease	Level of support for family and carers

Many of the intrinsic factors listed above are things that we are unable to influence. However, arguably, simple adjustments to extrinsic factors can contribute significantly to effective communication. Because Stans *et al.* (2013) argue that there is a lack of awareness and knowledge of communication vulnerability amongst health professionals, it is imperative that this is now prioritised in practice.

5.3 Communication vulnerability and ageing

The gradual decline in sensory and cognitive abilities has been described as an inevitability of normal ageing. While many older adults live healthy and active lives, with a great variation in how people age, it is also recognised that as people age, the prevalence of multiple chronic conditions increases (World Health Organization, 2015). Referred to as multimorbidity, the impact of the combined effects of each disorder can have a significant impact on function, quality of life and the individual's risk of mortality. With effective communication playing a central role in the process of adjusting and adapting to the ageing process, older adults who are communication vulnerable may be at particular risk.

Ageing and multimorbidity are also associated with increased use of healthcare provision, across a wide variety of clinical settings. As a nurse, you will be providing care for increasing numbers of older adults, many of whom will have complex care needs. An individual's ability to be understood, respected and responded to in a dignified manner is fundamental to the delivery of person-centred care. *Figure 5.1* outlines the consequences of ineffective communication.

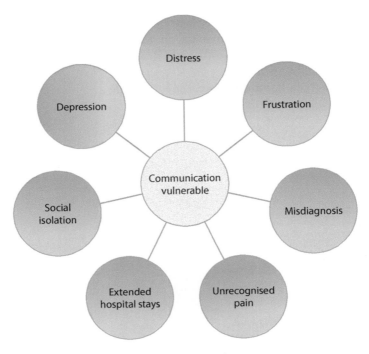

Figure 5.1 *The consequences of ineffective communication.*

Palmer *et al.* (2016) highlight that the ability to communicate effectively in older age is essential for:

- living independently
- pursuing personal goals and interests
- performing social roles and functions
- maintaining personal and familial relationships
- making decisions
- exercising control over quality of life and care.

Consider now the process of communication that was discussed in *Chapter 1*. In its simplistic form, communication can be defined as the sending and receiving of both verbal and non-verbal messages, between two or more people, and can be regarded as both a simple and a complex process. This is referred to as a linear model of communication and describes a process in which a sender transmits a message to a receiver:

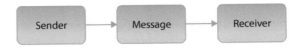

This linear model suggests that communication occurs in one direction only, with the sender responsible for not only the accuracy of the message, but also the tone. The receiver then interprets the verbal and/or non-verbal content of the message. However, the linear model assumes clarity of meaning and purpose of the message sent, and that the receiver is receptive, willing and able to receive and assimilate the message. However, Le May (2006) has highlighted that for a message to be effectively communicated it must be processed by a series of channels, which are listed in *Table 5.2*.

Table 5.2 *Examples of effective communication channels*

Communication channel	Example
Sensory	Hearing, seeing, touching, feeling, smelling, tasting
Motor	Speech, facial, expression, touch, gesture
Cognitive	Comprehension, memory, attention, thought, decision-making
Psychological functions	Emotional state, feelings
Social functions	Interpersonal relationships, expectations

Changes in one or more of these five communication channels will have an impact on communication, and the correlation between ageing and the disturbance of these channels is clear.

ACTIVITY 5.1

Think about a recent practice experience. Focus on an episode of care you provided for a patient.
- Reflect on any intrinsic factors the patient may have been experiencing that may have had an impact on the way they were able to communicate their needs.
- Now think of any extrinsic factors that may have impacted on effective communication.

Could anything have been altered to overcome any challenges encountered?

5.4 Sensory impairment

The World Health Organization identifies sensory impairment as among the major burdens of disability in older age, citing ageing as being associated with the decline of both auditory and visual function (World Health Organization, 2015).

In order to have a greater understanding of how we can support a person with sensory impairment, let us explore the impact of hearing and visual impairment, and deafblindness.

5.4.1 Hearing impairment

It is estimated that more than 70% of people over 70 years old in the UK have some degree of hearing impairment; this rises to 90% in people over 80 years old. As the population lives longer, the prevalence of impairment is estimated to increase by 14% each decade (Action on Hearing Loss, no date). Hearing impairment can have a significant impact on day-to-day activities, leading to depression, social withdrawal, confusion, miscommunication and increased risk of accidents.

There are three categories of hearing impairment and a number of reasons why a person may lose their hearing (*Table 5.3*). However, it is important to remember that hearing impairment is complex, and as such its symptoms will be experienced differently from one person to the next.

Table 5.3 *Hearing impairment: categories and causes*

Categories of hearing impairment
• Sensorineural hearing loss (inner ear)
• Conductive hearing loss (outer and middle ear)
• Mixed hearing loss – combination of sensorineural and conductive hearing loss

Causes of hearing loss
• Age-related damage to the cochlea (presbycusis) – difficulty in hearing high-frequency sounds
• Prolonged and repeated exposure to noise, e.g. in the workplace
• Genetic hearing loss
• Ototoxic drugs
• Tinnitus
• Impaction of cerumen (earwax)
• Infections
• Trauma

ACTIVITY 5.2

A patient has a moderate hearing impairment and has been admitted to A&E with shortness of breath.
- What are the background noises that may impact on their understanding of what is being said to them?
- How could this affect their care?

Blustein *et al.* (2018) believe that the impact of hearing impairment in clinical settings is often overlooked. Reflecting on *Activity 5.2*, you will recognise that hospitals can be noisy environments. The noise generated around the nurses' station, from telephones ringing, patient call bells, the clatter of trolleys, the alarm of infusion pumps, to the low hum of a pressure-relieving mattress, can be pervasive. Indeed, Pope *et al.* (2013) suggest that noise levels in hospitals can have a significant impact on a patient's ability to hear, understand and recall what is said to them by healthcare providers. This can lead to inequality of care, poor patient experience and significant costs to the NHS.

It is often assumed that an individual with age-related hearing loss has difficulty detecting sound; however, the difficulties often lie in the understanding, or intelligibility, of speech. Speech intelligibility is enhanced when the talker faces the listener, ensuring that their face and lips are visible, and gestures and facial expressions remain normal and are not exaggerated. In a noisy environment, we all have a tendency to shout, in an effort to make ourselves heard. However, raising the volume of the voice reduces clarity of speech, making it even more difficult to understand. Furthermore, raising the volume of the voice also adds to the cacophony of sound.

For many people with hearing impairments, the use of hearing aids can enhance the ability to comprehend speech and engage in conversation. However, for many people there is a reluctance to bring hearing aids into a clinical environment, fearing that these expensive and essential devices may get lost or broken. The simple initiative of introducing storage boxes for hearing aids, with information and tips on basic hearing aid maintenance and spare batteries, can be a positive measure in clinical practice, and something that should be encouraged.

Now let us look at what can be done to improve the quality of care received by patients who have hearing impairment. *Box 5.1* gives some strategies to promote effective communication with a person with hearing impairment.

BOX 5.1: COMMUNICATING WELL – HEARING IMPAIRMENT

- Ensure hearing impairment is recorded as part of the assessment and plan of care.
- Include details of type of hearing impairment. Is it unilateral or bilateral? Does the person lip read? Do they wear hearing aids?
- Avoid unnecessary noise (e.g. turn off TVs and radios, electric fans).
- Ensure adequate lighting.
- Gain the person's attention before speaking.
- Ensure that you are sitting face on to the person.
- Talk directly to the person, and avoid speaking to others at the same time.
- Do not cover your mouth when talking.
- Speak clearly, not too fast, and avoid over-enunciating words. Use normal lip movements and facial gestures.
- Avoid shouting as this will reduce clarity of speech.
- If necessary, repeat and/or rephrase.
- Hearing aids: If away from home environment, ensure safe storage. Ensure access to batteries and cleaning equipment.
- Encourage use of loop/telecoil system if available.
- Use electronic support devices where appropriate.
- Use British Sign Language (BSL).

5.4.2 Visual impairment

The Royal National Institute of Blind People estimates that 20% of adults over 75 years of age, and 50% of adults over 90 years, experience visual impairment (Royal National Institute of Blind People, 2018). Over 2 million people have a degree of impairment that results in significant impact on their daily lives. As with hearing, the prevalence of visual impairment is predicted to rise over the coming decades, doubling to over 4 million by 2050.

The main causes of visual impairment are listed below. With each condition affecting the ability to see and function in different ways it is important to remember, as with hearing impairment, that the effect of visual impairment will be unique to the individual.

- Uncorrected refractive error
- Age-related macular degeneration
- Cataract
- Glaucoma
- Diabetic eye disease.

The impact of visual impairment can be both debilitating and devastating, and coming to terms with the loss of sight can be difficult for both the individual and their families and carers. Thurston *et al.* (2010) describe those transitioning from sight to blindness as experiencing a profound sense of loss, similar to bereavement. The individual can experience low morale, feelings of depression, loneliness and isolation, and can withdraw from social contact. For older adults, vision loss may also occur at a time when other senses such as hearing and touch are also impaired, adding to a sense of isolation together with greater difficulties when performing activities of daily living.

ACTIVITY 5.3

Mary is 79 years old, and was diagnosed with type 2 diabetes 25 years ago. She has diabetic retinopathy and is registered as severely sight impaired. Mary has recently been experiencing symptoms related to peripheral vascular disease and has been referred to her local vascular specialist.

- Consider how her visual impairment may impact on her interaction with healthcare services.

Visual impairment can result in the individual encountering difficulties in accessing and negotiating healthcare services, and effective communication is essential to avoid this. Consideration must be given to both written and verbal communication. From the appointment letter that is sent through the post, written information about a procedure, signage in a hospital department, to the consent form and post-operative instructions, there is a reliance on the written word to disseminate information. Cupples *et al.* (2012) stress that the recognition that a person may have problems with their vision is essential for good healthcare.

There are several communication strategies that can be employed to support the person with visual impairments (see *Box 5.2*).

BOX 5.2: COMMUNICATING WELL – VISION IMPAIRMENT

- Ensure vision loss is recorded as part of assessment and plan of care.
- Ask the person to describe their level of vision, whether they require any help and what this might be.
- Does the person wear glasses? Do they have them at hand and are they the correct prescription? Is safe storage and cleaning equipment available?
- Poor lighting will be a barrier to communication for a person with visual impairment. Ensure the lighting is adequate, but also not too bright.
- Consider how you have positioned yourself in the room. Standing in front of a window will mean you may appear in silhouette with facial features hidden. If you are talking to a person with loss of central vision, they may prefer you to sit to one side of them. Conversely, place yourself directly in front of a person with loss of peripheral vision.
- Introduce others if in a group, and if you leave the room let the person know you are going.
- Describe what you are doing, or going to do, and any equipment you might be using.
- Make eye contact, even if this is not returned.
- Speak directly to the person, never speak via a third person.
- Try to avoid unnecessary background noise.
- Continue to use non-verbal communication; this will have a positive effect on the tone of your voice.

5.4.3 Deafblindness

Deafblindness is a term used to describe the impairment of both vision and hearing. Also referred to as dual sensory impairment, it is a condition found in all age groups, but the highest incidence is amongst older adults. A person is regarded as deafblind if, together, their visual and hearing impairments cause difficulties with communication, access to information and mobility. The Department of Health has published useful guidance on this issue (Department of Health, 2014).

It is important to acknowledge that whilst the term deafblind does indeed describe a person with no functional hearing or vision, many people who are deafblind have some degree of sight and hearing. In this instance, it is therefore important to help maximise the potential of the less impaired sense, using the strategies listed in *Boxes 5.1* and *5.2*. When there is significant loss in both senses it is essential that the person is supported in finding alternative communication methods, for example the deafblind manual alphabet, and portable listening devices.

5.5 **Aphasia**

Take a moment to think about the last time you interacted with someone. It may have been saying goodbye to family members this morning, in the coffee shop queue this afternoon, or speaking with someone at the train station. Maybe you sent a quick text message to a friend, or an email to a colleague.

Whatever the interaction was, it was likely that you used a series of gestures, facial expressions and words to express yourself. Maybe you used an emoji or two within the text message. You will also have needed to interpret the other person's gestures, expressions and words to make sense of what they were saying.

For many individuals, changes in the way spoken and written language is processed mean that interpretation of these interactions can be significantly impaired. This is referred to as aphasia. Aphasia is an acquired language disorder, resulting in damage to the speech and language centres of the brain, and can be a direct result of:

- cerebral vascular accident (CVA)
- traumatic brain injury
- brain tumour
- progressive neurological condition.

While any of the above can lead to aphasia, a CVA is the most common cause. It is estimated that around a third of people who have a CVA will also experience aphasia. However, Thompson and McKeever (2014) highlight that care after stroke can often focus on the physiological event rather than the patient's experience of aphasia.

Aphasia may affect the person's ability to express themselves and also to comprehend speech, affecting their ability to talk and write, and in turn to understand spoken or written language. Processing information, thinking, memory, problem-solving and reasoning may also be impacted.

There are different classifications of aphasia, as shown in *Table 5.4*.

Table 5.4 *Classification of aphasia*

Type of aphasia	Experience and impact
Expressive (or Broca's aphasia)	• Caused by injury to the left frontal regions of the brain • Difficulty with **producing** language, both spoken and written • Comprehension relatively unaffected • Difficulty finding the right words, and forming sentences
Receptive (or Wernicke's aphasia)	• Caused by injury to the left temporal region of the brain • Difficulty with **understanding** language, both spoken and written • Production of speech relatively unaffected • Sentences are fluent but often contain non-existent or irrelevant words • There is little awareness that the sentence does not make sense
Global	• Caused by injury to multiple areas of the brain • Difficulty both **producing** and **understanding** language, both spoken and written

Aphasia can affect the quantity and quality of daily interactions, quality of life and psychological wellbeing. It can also affect family members and have an impact on relationships. *Figure 5.2* illustrates the impact of aphasia.

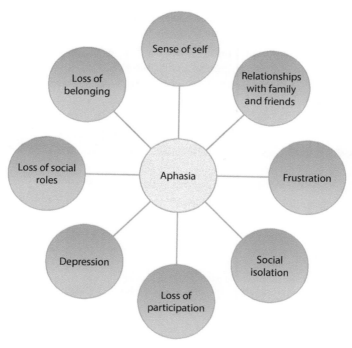

Figure 5.2 *The impact of aphasia.*

During your practice placements you may have cared for a patient who has experienced a CVA, or you may have discussed a similar scenario as part of your nursing studies.

Reflecting on the potential care needs of a patient who has experienced a CVA, consider the specific communication challenges that may be experienced by this patient. Can you list some of the specific problems they may have?

It is recognised that many people who experience a CVA, and are experiencing aphasia, also have a visual and/or hearing impairment.

Consider the additional challenges this would present to both the patient and their family.

It is accepted that successful communication depends on both the skill and experience of the person with aphasia and the skill and experience of the conversation partner. Training for family members to support them in their role of conversation partner is fundamental. However, it is also essential to recognise that nurses may also lack the knowledge, skill and confidence required to facilitate conversation with a person who has aphasia. The focus of communication between nurse and patient can often be on the nursing task in hand, the practical and technical, with little importance placed on getting to know the patient through dialogue. This then creates an imbalance, and one in which the patient feels disempowered and is unable to participate in their own care.

There are several strategies designed to reduce barriers to communication, allowing individuals with aphasia to express their needs. These are listed in *Box 5.3*. It must be acknowledged that involving family and friends as advocates, as a source of knowledge about the individual, can be a valuable strategy. However, caution must be exercised, as this may increase the risk of misinterpretation and have further impact on the individual's autonomy.

BOX 5.3: COMMUNICATING WELL – APHASIA

- Ensure background noise is kept to a minimum.
- Focus sentences on one idea at a time, using short clear sentences.
- Ask closed questions, requiring only a yes/no response. If this is not possible, offer only two choices.
- Clarify and rephrase if necessary.
- Do not rush; take time for the person with aphasia to respond. Don't answer, or finish sentences for them.
- Be alert to signs of miscomprehension, and modify the question if necessary.
- Introduce gestures, e.g. thumbs up and down, head nodding, enhanced facial expressions.
- Establish how the person uses a limited vocabulary – are there phrases that are often used to indicate agreement?
- Use of augmentative and alternative communication aids, e.g. gesturing, body language, paper and pen, picture boards or high-tech computerised systems.

5.6 Dementia

Nurses provide care for people with dementia in a variety of clinical settings, including hospitals, care homes and the person's own home. It is estimated that around 60% of people receiving support from home care services are living with dementia (UK Homecare Association, 2013), whilst 25% of hospital beds are occupied by people with dementia. Admission to hospital is often a result of a physical illness, rather than dementia, and the patient's diagnosis of dementia is often overlooked. Consequently, the length of stay for these patients is often longer and the outcomes poorer. Admission to any healthcare setting can be a frightening and confusing experience, and skilful and sensitive communication skills are fundamental if a person with dementia is to receive high-quality, person-centred care. An understanding of dementia and the impact it has on both the person and their family is essential.

Dementia is a term used to define a range of conditions that affect the brain and result in overall functional impairment. A person may experience a collection of symptoms including memory loss, problems with perception, reasoning and communication skills, and difficulties with activities of daily living.

There are two websites you may find it useful to access: www.alzheimers.org.uk for further information about the types of dementia and its symptoms, and www.alzheimersresearchuk.org/about-dementia/facts-stats for statistics about the prevalence of dementia.

In a drive to improve hospital care for people with dementia, the Royal College of Nursing has published its five SPACE principles of good dementia care (Royal College of Nursing, 2011). These are listed here, but you can also access them at www.rcn.org. uk/clinical-topics/dementia/current-work:

- Staff who are skilled and have time to care
- Partnership working with carers
- Assessment and early identification of people living with dementia
- Care plans that are person-centred and individualised
- Environments that are dementia friendly

The aim of the five principles is to ensure appropriate delivery of care, and you will see that underpinning each is effective communication.

So how does dementia affect a person's ability to communicate effectively? Dementia is a condition that affects expressive and receptive language abilities, with the decline in the ability to communicate effectively usually progressive and gradual. However, it is also recognised that communication impairment in people with dementia varies greatly, and the importance of patient involvement in assessment, planning and decision-making is paramount for person-centred care.

A person with dementia may:

- have trouble finding the right word (aphasia)
- find it difficult to understand what is being said
- repeat words, phrases and ideas, with lack of coherence or logic in speech
- become 'stuck' on certain sounds
- experience difficulty recognising familiar objects, people, sights, places and sounds (agnosia)
- have a decreased attention span.

Because dementia is a condition that is associated with ageing, a person with dementia is also often living with other sensory impairments, for example visual and hearing. This can further impact on communication, leading to loss of confidence, anxiety, depression and social withdrawal. An inability to communicate using words may then lead to behaviour that others perceive as unusual or uncharacteristic, with frustration being exhibited by verbal and physical aggression, and withdrawal. Referred to as resistiveness to care, this is often the only way the person can communicate their unmet needs.

ACTIVITY 5.5

Reflect on a previous episode of care for a person with dementia – maybe when you were carrying out an assessment, or assisting the patient with personal hygiene.

- Did you adapt the words you used?
- What tone and volume did you use?
- If you were working alongside a colleague how did they communicate with the person? Did you recognise a change in words used, or tone?
- Consider how you adapted your non-verbal communication.

We recognise that the words used, and the tone and volume of speech, become increasingly important when communicating with a person with dementia. Research suggests there is a correlation between emotional tone used by healthcare professionals, and resistiveness to care behaviours (Williams and Herman, 2011). Emotional tone refers to changes in pitch, loudness and speech rate, and conveys different emotion. A manifestation of this is elderspeak, a modification of speech that results in a patronising and infantilising communication approach. Identified as a common intergeneration style of communication, modifications such as child-like speech, inappropriate terms of endearment such as 'honey' and 'sweetheart', and the use of collective pronouns are used. Examples of this might be "It is time we had a bath, isn't it?"

Now consider that you have found the right words, you have adopted the correct tone, but your facial expression and posture communicate lack of interest and irritation. You may be standing over the person and letting your gaze drift, rather than sitting opposite and establishing eye contact. This non-verbal communication, which includes body movement, posture, touch and gesture, helps to communicate attitude and feelings. For communication to be effective both verbal and non-verbal communication must support each other.

When a person with dementia is being cared for at home, they are surrounded by information that tells us who they are, their culture, their role within the family, their personality, hobbies and interests. Once in a hospital or a care home setting this point of reference, for both the person and the healthcare professional, is lost. The creation of a life history record, whether in the form of a 'This is me' booklet, collage or photograph album, provides a valuable insight into the person as an individual and enhances person-centred care. By involving family and friends in documenting the person's family and cultural background, routines and preferences, effective communication can be supported. *Box 5.4* shows some further strategies to support effective communication between the nurse and the person with dementia.

BOX 5.4: COMMUNICATING WELL – DEMENTIA

- Find a space to talk, where there is minimal ambient noise and distractions. Move to a more suitable area if necessary. Is there any background noise that can be minimised? For example, can the television or radio be turned off? Do you need to shut a window to block out noise from traffic?
- Ensure good lighting. Provide adjustable lighting that can be adapted to the situation. Use natural lighting where possible.
- Ensure privacy. Can this conversation be overheard?
- Position yourself so you are each on the same level, as this will facilitate the interpretation of body language.
- If the person has a visual and/or hearing impairment as well, consider the strategies in *Boxes 5.1* and *5.2*.

BOX 5.4: COMMUNICATING WELL – DEMENTIA (*continued*)

- Before starting a conversation, gently gain the person's attention. Is this the right time for this interaction? Is the person tired? Does the person have any pain that needs to be managed before the interaction can take place? Are there visitors present?
- Use the person's preferred name and introduce yourself.
- Take time to find out something about the person. Do they have a life history record?
- If the interaction is taking place with a family member or carer also present, ensure that the person with dementia is included and not ignored.
- Keep sentences simple and short. As a person's dementia progresses, the processing of information will take longer. Take time to communicate and wait for a response.
- Use closed questions, i.e. those that require just a yes or no response.
- Consider the emotional tone you are using and avoid elderspeak.
- Listen – effective communication is not just about speaking.

5.7 Breaking bad news

Nurses often find themselves in situations in which they are required to break bad news to patients and their loved ones. Breaking bad news is a complex activity and, if done badly, can cause detrimental effects on both the patient and those close to them. It can impact negatively on the relationship between patient and health professional, and the patient's long-term memory of that episode of their lives. Conversely, if done well it can help build a sense of trust and openness, strengthen the therapeutic relationship, and help facilitate coping.

ACTIVITY 5.6

The way in which you are involved in breaking bad news will be dependent on your role and the clinical setting you work in. Discuss with your supervisors their experiences of breaking bad news. Take a moment to consider any episodes you have observed, or been involved in, relating to breaking bad news.
- What were the main things you learned from your discussions?
- If you have observed or been involved in breaking bad news, how did you feel during the experience and after?

Bad, sad or significant news, in relation to a patient's health, has the capacity to turn the expectations and perceptions of present and future upside down. When we refer to bad news, there is a tendency to focus on those conversations that may involve a life-limiting or terminal diagnosis. However, it is important to recognise the variety of conversations nurses may have with patients, and their family or friends, that may elicit reactions of distress.

Warnock (2014) considers the breaking of bad news to be a process rather than a one-off event. It involves helping the patient to prepare for, then receive and process, and ultimately cope with the news they are given. This could be at the time of a diagnosis of a life-limiting or life-changing condition, when treatment options have changed, or when informing relatives and loved ones of a patient's death.

In these situations, it is essential that the nurse demonstrates both effective and compassionate communication skills.

However, the term 'bad news' can be subjective and as such it is important that the nurse does not make assumptions regarding how a person may react. What we may perceive as 'bad news' for a patient may actually be a relief. A patient may have had troubling and painful symptoms for a while, undergone a variety of diagnostic tests, and spent many weeks wondering what was wrong. With a firm diagnosis, they may now feel they are able to make informed decisions about their treatment and make appropriate plans for their future. In contrast, a patient given a diagnosis of type 2 diabetes may suddenly feel apprehensive about the long-term implications for employment and financial support.

Warnock *et al.* (2010) identify the following barriers nurses experience when breaking bad news:

- Lack of time
- The patient not wanting to know
- Feeling unprepared when the issue arose unexpectedly
- Barriers to communication (e.g. language, aphasia)
- Lack of information
- Patient not being told at relative's request
- Lack of privacy
- Verbal or physical abuse from patient/relative
- Not believing this is a nurse's role.

It is argued that while guidelines exist for the breaking of bad news during pre-planned consultations, where information about diagnosis, prognosis and treatment is often shared with patients and their family, in reality the process of breaking bad news is often ongoing and may involve multiple interactions with different healthcare staff (Warnock *et al.*, 2010).

Let us finally return to *Activity 5.6*, and consider the moment the person received the bad news. As a nurse, you may have been in the consulting room, or you may have been sitting with the patient later. The patient may have asked you to clarify what had been said earlier as they didn't quite understand the terminology. You may have been a student with a community nurse who, when visiting a patient, was asked by family members "How long has Dad got left?". You may have been helping a patient get dressed when they ask if the weakness in their right arm will ever improve. These incidents would have probably been unexpected and you will not have time to prepare an answer. This illustrates the unique position nurses are in, and the importance of skilful and sensitive communication. *Box 5.5* provides you with some strategies to support this unique position.

BOX 5.5: COMMUNICATING WELL – BREAKING BAD NEWS

- Consider who needs to be present during this conversation. Does a family member/friend need to be there to provide support and facilitate understanding?
- Is there anyone present who may be communication vulnerable? If so, consider the specific strategies of communicating well, previously explored in this chapter, when breaking bad news.
- Ensure an environment that is private, and where interruptions can be minimised. Is it a comfortable environment where everyone present can sit?
- If the conversation is planned, do you have all the relevant information you need? Consider how you are going to deliver the news; what words and phrases are you going to use? Avoid the use of jargon and euphemisms that may be misunderstood or misinterpreted.
- Do not make assumptions about what the person and family already know – seek clarification of this.
- When providing information, ensure it is accurate and clear. Be honest but also offer encouragement, hope and support.
- Use open-ended questions, which allow the person to respond to questions in more detail and help to clarify understanding.
- Allow time for questions and explanations.
- Do not try to fill silences – the person may need this time to process the news given.
- Expect an emotional reaction, and allow time for this. However, also remember that people respond to the breaking of bad news in different ways.
- Provide written information if available.
- As part of the conversation, agree a plan of what will happen next. Will there be a follow-up appointment, or a chance to continue the discussion at another time? Ensure that the person and family have a sense of control and know what to expect next.
- If the conversation is unplanned, listen to the concerns of the person. Do not provide answers if you do not have them, but reassure the person that you will seek out the information they require or refer them to someone who may be able to help.
- The breaking of bad news can also impact on the emotional wellbeing of the nurse. Take time to reflect on episodes of care when you are involved in the breaking of bad news, and seek support from team members and the support mechanisms within your organisation.

CASE STUDY

You have recently started a new post on an acute stroke unit. It is 07:30 and you have just arrived on shift. During the night Barbara Powell, a 73-year-old woman, was admitted to the ward after collapsing at home. A CT scan was performed an hour after admission and she has been diagnosed as having had a CVA, with damage to the left frontal region of the brain. Barbara is now receiving care in the four-bedded high dependency care bay on the ward. As she is awaiting assessment of her swallow reflex, she is currently nil by mouth. She has intravenous fluids *in situ*, and these are being administered via an infusion pump.

Barbara has a history of age-related macular degeneration and has recently been fitted with hearing aids for bilateral hearing impairment.

CASE STUDY (*continued*)

■ Consider the intrinsic and extrinsic factors that will have an impact on communication.

That morning you spend time with Barbara, you assess her activities of daily living in order to make a systematic nursing diagnosis, identify person-centred goals and initiate a plan of care. It quickly becomes apparent that Barbara is finding it difficult to find the right words and form sentences. She appears to understand speech, but uses the same repetitive phrase "and then" in response. This is frustrating for her and she is very tearful.

■ Reflecting back on this chapter, what type of aphasia is Barbara experiencing?

The next day Barbara has been transferred to a bed on the main ward. It is visiting time. Barbara is married to Clive, and they have recently celebrated their 50th wedding anniversary. They have two sons, Nigel and John. Barbara has always taken an active role in the care of her three grandchildren, and regularly collects them from school and takes them home for tea. The eldest of her three grandchildren, Isaac, aged 14, is keen to visit his grandmother in hospital. He has arrived with his father Nigel. Clive is also visiting.

■ What strategies can you adopt to facilitate effective communication for Barbara and her family?

■ Consider the advice and support you can provide the family.

■ How would you structure a plan of care which focuses on Barbara's communication needs?

Summary

The correlation between ageing and multimorbidity is recognised, and effective communication plays a central role in adjustment and adaptation to the ageing process. As the ageing population grows, the number of those who are communication vulnerable will increase. Nurses have a duty of care to ensure that the needs of both patients and their families are safeguarded, and that provision of high-quality, person-centred and therapeutic care is maintained. Effective communication between the patient who is communication vulnerable and the nurse is influenced by a number of intrinsic and extrinsic factors. Whilst the intrinsic factors are largely beyond our control, we are able to influence the extrinsic factors. Often small alterations can have a significant impact on the care that patients, their families and carers receive and experience.

KEY LEARNING POINTS

Four key points to take away from *Chapter 5*:

☑ Communication vulnerability is on the increase and has a significant impact on how people experience healthcare.

☑ Holistic assessment of the intrinsic factors that may mean a person is communication vulnerable is essential to the planning and implementation of person-centred care.

☑ Take time to consider whether simple adjustments to the environment may have a positive impact on effective communication.

☑ Become an ambassador for people who are communication vulnerable within your workplace, and raise the profile of the challenge they face.

FURTHER READING

Buckman, R. (1992) *How to Break Bad News: a guide for health care professionals.* The John Hopkins University Press.

National Institute for Health and Care Excellence (2013) *Stroke rehabilitation in adults.* CG162. Section 1.8: Communication. Available at: www.nice. org.uk/guidance/cg162/resources/stroke-rehabilitation-in-adults-pdf-35109688408261 (accessed 19 July 2019).

NHS (2018) *Dementia guide. Communicating with someone with dementia.* Available at: www.nhs.uk/conditions/dementia/communication-and-dementia (accessed 19 July 2019).

REFERENCES

Action on Hearing Loss (no date). *Facts and figures.* Available at: www. actiononhearingloss.org.uk/about-us/our-research-and-evidence/facts-and-figures (accessed 19 July 2019).

Blustein, J., Weinstein, B.E., Chodosh, J. and Freeman, M.L. (2018) Tackling hearing loss to improve the care of older adults. *British Medical Journal,* **360**: k21.

Cupples, M., Hart, P., Johnston, A. and Jackson, A.J. (2012) Improving healthcare access for people with visual impairment and blindness. *British Medical Journal,* **344**: e542.

Dart, A.M. (2011) *Motivational Interviewing in Nursing Practice: empowering the patient.* Jones & Bartlett Learning.

Department of Health (2014) *Care and Support for Deafblind Children and Adults Policy Guidance.* Available at: https://assets.publishing.service.gov. uk/government/uploads/system/uploads/attachment_data/file/388198/ Care_and_Support_for_Deafblind_Children_and_Adults_Policy_ Guidance_12_12_14_FINAL.pdf (accessed 19 July 2019).

Department of Health (2015) *No Secrets: guidance on developing and implementing multi-agency policies and procedures to protect vulnerable adults from abuse.* Available at: www.gov.uk/government/publications/no-secrets-guidance-on-protecting-vulnerable-adults-in-care (accessed 19 July 2019).

Green, D. (2015) Safeguarding and protection of vulnerable adults. *Nursing and Residential Care,* **17(5)**: 293–6.

Le May, A.C. (2006) *Communication challenges and skills,* in Redfern, S.J. and Ross, F.M. (eds) *Nursing Older People.* Elsevier Churchill Livingstone, pp. 166–7.

Nursing and Midwifery Council (2018) *The Code: professional standards of practice and behaviour for nurses, midwives and nursing associates*. NMC. Available at: www.nmc.org.uk/globalassets/sitedocuments/nmc-publications/nmc-code.pdf (accessed 19 July 2019).

Palmer, A.D., Newsom, J.T. and Rook, K.S. (2016) How does difficulty communicating affect the social relationships of older adults? An exploration using data from a national survey. *Journal of Communication Disorders*, **62**: 131–46.

Pope, D.S., Gallun, F.J. and Kampel, S. (2013) Effect of hospital noise on patients' ability to hear, understand, and recall speech. *Research in Nursing & Health*, **36(3)**: 228–41.

Price, B. (2017) Developing patient rapport, trust and therapeutic relationships. *Nursing Standard*, **31(50)**: 52–63.

Royal College of Nursing (2011) *Dementia: commitment to the care of people with dementia in hospital settings*. Available at: www.rcn.org.uk/professional-development/publications/pub-004235 (accessed 19 July 2019).

Royal National Institute of Blind People (2018) Eye health and sight loss stats and facts. Available at: www.rnib.org.uk/sites/default/files/Eye%20health%20and%20sight%20loss%20stats%20and%20facts.pdf (accessed 19 July 2019).

Stans, S.E., Dalemans, R., de Witte, L. and Beurskens, A. (2013) Challenges in the communication between 'communication vulnerable' people and their social environment: an exploratory qualitative study. *Patient Education and Counselling*, **92(3)**: 302–12.

Thompson, J. and McKeever, M. (2014) The impact of stroke aphasia on health and well-being and appropriate nursing interventions: an exploration using the Theory of Human Scale Development. *Journal of Clinical Nursing*, **23(3–4)**, 410–20.

Thurston, M., Thurston, A. and McLeod, J. (2010) Socio-economic effects of the transition from sight to blindness. *The British Journal of Visual Impairment*, **28(2)**: 90–112.

UK Homecare Association (2013) *UKHCA Dementia Strategy and Plan*. Available at: www.ukhca.co.uk/pdfs/UKHCADementiaStrategy201202final.pdf (accessed 19 July 2019).

Warnock, C. (2014) Breaking bad news: issues relating to nursing practice. *Nursing Standard*, **28(45)**: 51–8.

Warnock, C., Tod, A., Foster, J. and Soreny, C. (2010) Breaking bad news in inpatient clinical settings: role of the nurse. *Journal of Advanced Nursing*, **66(7)**: 1543–55.

Williams, K.N. and Herman, R.E. (2011) Linking resident behavior to dementia care communication: effects of emotional tone. *Behavior Therapy*, **42(1)**: 42–6.

World Health Organization (2015) *World Report on Ageing and Health.* Available at: https://apps.who.int/iris/bitstream/handle/10665/186463/9789240694811_eng.pdf?sequence=1 (accessed 19 July 2019).

Chapter 6
Communication and diversity

Naomi A. Watson

LEARNING OUTCOMES

By the end of this chapter you should be able to:

6.1 Recognise diversity and its globalised, localised, social and contextual relevance to your communication practice

6.2 Appreciate the impact of culture, religion, ethnicity, sexuality and other forms of diversity, and the intersectional nature of their effects on patients

6.3 Understand interprofessional and intercultural language barrier dilemmas experienced by some staff and patients

6.4 Have an awareness of your role in advancing communication in diversity in the workplace and the possible impact and implications of unconscious bias

6.5 Support colleagues, peers, patients and service users to develop better skills for communicating effectively by addressing discriminatory practice through diversity championing, and reflective practice.

6.1 Introduction

This chapter will explore communication in diversity and consider how you can develop and enhance skills to benefit patients and their carers and families. Good communication skills are an integral aspect of practising safely and effectively as a nurse. Patients, families and carers depend on you to help them understand and navigate the complexities of the healthcare environment, which is usually a stressful and frightening experience for them. This is even more relevant if they have social, cultural, physical and/or linguistic needs that could limit their understanding and make it difficult for them to keep up with events relating to their care, or to articulate their care needs. Understanding how to effectively communicate in diverse populations and in a culturally competent manner is an ethical requirement and is covered by all healthcare regulatory bodies in their professional standards and codes.

Within the NMC *Code*, section 1.3 states "avoid making assumptions and recognise diversity and individual choice" and section 7.3 states "use a range of verbal and non-verbal communication methods, and consider cultural sensitivities, to better understand and respond to people's personal and health needs" (Nursing and Midwifery Council, 2018).

For all patients, regardless of their culture, ethnicity or physical condition, being unable to make themselves understood may make them fearful and anxious, which could further trigger other negative outcomes in health and social care. This runs the risk of compromising their safe recovery from illness, or the achievement of positive outcomes. As you develop and improve your understanding of how to effectively communicate in diversity, it is imperative that you critically reflect regularly as part of your learning so you can enhance this important skill and share with your peers and colleagues.

6.2 **Embracing diversity**

Access to the internet has contributed to social and economic globalisation. This is structured around varied methods of digital and other communication, including electronic media. An increasing number of people worldwide are now connected through media such as Facebook, Twitter and Instagram, and by continuing movement of people through migration or vacation. Communication is unintentionally much more complex, affecting all societies, including the UK. Nurses have to recognise diversity, and contribute towards promoting and respecting diverse communities, both locally and globally. To contribute effectively, you must demonstrate a commitment to adapting the way you communicate in different contexts.

Whether as part of a multidisciplinary team (MDT) meeting, informing a group of family members when breaking bad news, gathering information for an assessment in order to plan and deliver care, or performing a nursing task that needs to be carefully explained to a patient, there is a requirement to ensure that every individual who is different is catered for within their specific socially diverse context. English-speaking patients with certain types of physical and/or psychological health conditions may have difficulty expressing their wishes. As a multicultural society, the UK is made up of diverse groups with many social and cultural perspectives (Holland and Hogg, 2010), even among those who speak English. Patient and service user populations continue to diversify in line with social structures overall (Office for National Statistics, 2012).

In order to reduce well-documented health inequalities and healthcare disparities, UK policy-makers continue to stress the requirement that services should be sensitive to the needs of service users and their carers (Equality and Human Rights Commission, 2013).

ACTIVITY 6.1

Spend some time thinking about the types of people you meet daily, first, in your practice, then in your local area/region/community.

To what extent do you think your local demographic cohort/s reflect the diverse UK society as a whole? How are they different from you?

Which differences are you comfortable with, or specifically find problematic?

Think about possible actions (at least one) that you can take to show your awareness of the importance of embracing diversity, both at work and in the community.

Now that you have had time to think about the make-up of people locally and at work in terms of their diversity, you may have been able to work through your own thoughts on the matter and how it relates to you as an individual. If you are in a rural part of the country, you may meet many older people, and if you are in or near a large city, you may have come across a more diverse group of people. It is perhaps inevitable that your personal comfort zone would be challenged, depending on the people you meet and interact with. For example, some people may find it easy to talk to, and interact with, older people, but feel less confident in communicating with younger people or people who have a mental health condition. Others struggle to talk to people who only speak very little English, while some may not know what to say to a young adolescent person who may be experiencing difficulty in understanding their sexuality.

You may have identified one or more possible actions that you could take to show your willingness to embrace the diversity around you. The fact that you are engaging with this chapter could indicate you are ready to learn more about communication in diversity and could serve as your first possible action. Another possible follow-up action could be to arrange a discussion with your supervisor or colleague in order to plan and undertake a difficult communication session with any clients/patients in your own area, whether it is older people, younger patients, patients with different cultural backgrounds, a patient with an autistic spectrum disorder, or someone with a mental health condition. Your supervisor could support you by giving you guidance where possible.

Bramhall (2014) suggests one of the challenges with communication generally in the health workplace is the negative impact of a lack of time and privacy in a busy health environment. This is even more significant during episodes of communication with diverse patients. Talking with your supervisor could help you to plan and set up a communication session in advance, at a time and place that will be conducive to optimising a positive outcome from the encounter. This could significantly improve your learning, knowledge and skills. Additionally, reducing the use of phrases and slang with which patients are not familiar and should not be expected to understand is another way of showing a willingness to embrace diversity. This is never an easy one to achieve as the use of jargon and abbreviations is commonplace and taken for granted in the health workplace.

6.3 In what ways are we diverse?

6.3.1 Culture

Culture is a widely used term, generally considered to be a set of beliefs or specific traditions and general values which are held by, and used to identify, individuals and/or groups in their social environment (Holland and Hogg, 2010). When it is identified within this context, it may sometimes fail to recognise the fluidity of some cultural norms, or the ability of individuals to locate themselves across cultures. Recognising culture from individual and not just group or cohort beliefs and perspectives helps to provide a wider basis of understanding that cohort groups are not necessarily homogenous. This fosters a more appropriate way of identifying health and communication needs. The emphasis here is on ensuring that you communicate using a person-centred approach rather than make any assumptions because individuals belong to a particular group. However, it is also important to be aware of the cultural implications of issues such as therapeutic touch and non-verbal cues of communication when working with some culturally diverse patients (Crisp and Meleady, 2012).

6.3.2 Religion

Globalised societies have diverse and varied belief systems and you will come across some, or many, in your healthcare working environment. Many are generally well known, such as Christianity, Islam, Buddhism, Judaism and Sikhism, for example, but you may encounter many others.

Religious beliefs may at times interfere with the type of care that a patient requires, especially where it restricts its followers from participating in certain types of medical procedures, such as organ donation or giving and receiving blood. For example, Jehovah's Witnesses (JW) who present themselves and maybe their children for medical care could have very strong views about accepting blood and blood products. This is now quite widely known in healthcare practice, and could at times present some dilemmas in care. Your supervisor can be a helpful support to enable you to understand and navigate any communication with JW patients, their children and other family members. As a student or registered practitioner, it is still required that you recognise the need to treat all diverse patients sensitively and with respect, seeking at all times to provide them with alternative treatment options where there are objections to a particular care regime.

Understanding and respecting the belief systems and religion of patients and service users helps in ensuring successful care outcomes and reduces conflicts in care management and communication. It helps to recognise that belief systems are personal and must be discussed with individual patients with care, without necessarily thinking that one has to agree or disagree with the other's beliefs.

Where there are very strong views or disagreement, this can be discussed with your supervisor prior to an episode of care for a particular patient.

6.3.3 Ethnicity

Ethnicity is a broad concept that refers to a social group with a shared cultural, historical, geographical, linguistic and/or religious tradition that distinguishes it from other groups.

According to the Office for National Statistics (2012) there is an increase in ethnic diversity in the population of England and Wales. London was reported to be the most diverse area, while Wales was the least diverse. The ONS also reported a reduction in the percentage of the white population from 94.1% in 1991 to 86% in 2011. Possible reasons for this could be migration and people movement, or reporting patterns in the census. The new census, due in 2021, will most likely provide a clearer overview of diversity across the UK. However, over the previous two decades there has been an upward shift in population demographics in terms of ethnicity. Additions to this shift have included not only refugees and asylum seekers but Eastern and Western European migration.

Figure 6.1 shows the percentage population estimates for the various minority ethnic groups in England and Wales that the Office for National Statistics identifies, based on the census in 2011, excluding White British who made up 80.5% of the total population. It shows great and increasing diversity in the ethnic composition of our society (ONS, 2012).

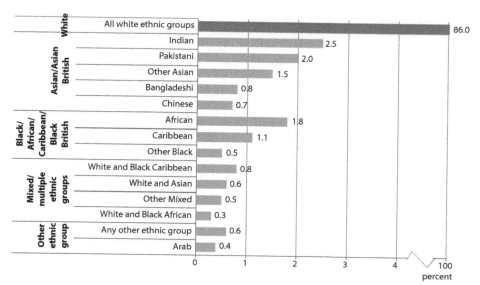

Figure 6.1 *Ethnic groups, 2001–2011, England and Wales (ONS, 2012).*
Notes:
1. Comparability issues exist between these ethnic groups for the 2001 and 2011 Census.
2. No comparable data exists for these ethnic groups in the 2001 Census.

We have looked at population statistics (*Figure 6.1*) to help you appreciate diversity in our society. An understanding of the population ethnic mix should contribute to planning strategies that will help to improve communication among all groups in healthcare. Unless a planned strategy is used it will be much more difficult to achieve care that is culturally competent. The emphasis is on our recognition of the impact of stereotypical assumptions and actions on diverse patients in our care, and begins with your own awareness and action (Sleek, 2018).

6.3.4 Sexual orientation

It is now an expectation that those who provide nursing and care services recognise their responsibilities towards people of varied sexual orientation, including lesbian, gay, bisexual, transgender and queer people (LGBTQ). The Equality Act (2010) gives every individual the right to be treated with respect regardless of their declared gender status. The emerging research also identifies a growing awareness of the gender debate, including the right of individuals to choose if and when they wish to declare their status.

The evidence has also identified that LGBTQ people experience disparities in healthcare, especially relating to communication (Borschman and Marino, 2019). Recent research suggests that LGBTQ young people and adolescents are at a very high risk of self-harming, feeling misunderstood and excluded, and the numbers experiencing depression are increasing. The evidence also suggests that there has been an increase in the number of adolescents who have attempted suicide because of issues relating to sexuality and sexual orientation (Irish *et al.*, 2018).

Preparation and training for delivering care is a requirement that should not be taken for granted, given the likely challenges that may arise. As a student, your supervisor, senior colleagues or diversity champion within your organisation will be able to support you when working with any patients in the above categories. As with all aspects of diverse communications, there is a requirement to engage with your personal responsibilities as someone who provides services to the general public, to be fair and supportive regardless of personal views, and to seek help if you have any difficulties providing care because of your own values/beliefs/conscience or any other challenges.

Becoming aware of any possible unconscious bias (discussed later in this chapter) and understanding how this may affect the way you deliver care to individuals is a first step in being able to work effectively with all LGBTQ patients. As a student, you may also be required to support those who may need help in coming to terms with their decisions to become known (coming out) in terms of their sexual orientation. Some adolescents and young people may ask for help and guidance, for example to approach their parents. Others may also need support with their mental health where they are trying to navigate personal dilemmas of sexual identity, biological health and gender differentiation and confusion as young adults.

To provide effective care, nurses and healthcare workers must communicate with sensitivity and inclusive respect, making sure that they ask each individual their status and preferences instead of relying on assumptions about the sexuality of any individual (Borschman and Marino, 2019).

ACTIVITY 6.2

Think about an episode of care in which you had to care for a patient who declared themselves to be any one or more of the following:

Transgender person, persons who practised varying religions (e.g. Jehovah's Witness, Christianity, Islam, Buddhism, Sikhism, Hinduism, Jewish orthodox, Rastafarianism), a homosexual male, a gay female, a black, Asian and minority ethnic (BAME) disabled man/woman. Think of your initial feelings about the patient.

What were the issues for you that could interfere with your care for that patient (i.e. relating to diet, medical treatment, physical/personal care, care of the dying, last offices care, use of ward toilets/bathrooms, etc.)?

Was the episode of care straightforward? Write down any awkward moments in the care encounter.

Was the patient happy with their care or able to express their views?

How did you negotiate the required care for each individual?

If you are comfortable doing so, share your thoughts with a colleague or peer.

What did you learn about the episode of care that will help you for future episodes of care?

6.3.5 Age

Working and communicating with older people can be challenging if you do not have the knowledge and skills to deliver effective person-centred care. It is important that older people do not feel patronised and they should be treated with dignity at all times. You will need to talk to people individually when possible, ensuring that you know what their wishes are in terms of how they want to be addressed, and their preferences for diet, hygiene requirements and social needs, rather than making assumptions because they are older. Dignity in care is very important for all patients; for older patients who may be vulnerable, this is paramount.

6.3.6 Language

Although the UK is mainly English-speaking, our society is as diversely multilingual as it is multicultural. There are well over 100 different languages spoken daily, not just by migrant communities but also by regional communities and in Wales, Northern Ireland and Scotland (ONS, 2012). Some languages are more prevalent than others, for example the main European languages such as French, Spanish and German, but they all present challenges. Language barriers have always been recognised as a major cause of disparities in healthcare, especially care in an acute care setting, which could compromise patient safety (Hull, 2016; Rein, 2016).

Below are some simple strategies you can adopt when working with and caring for people from culturally and linguistically diverse backgrounds (adapted from the New South Wales Department of Education and Training, 2009):

- Consider your choice of language and the words you use. Some idioms or slang language may not be understood by people from another linguistic background (or people within the same linguistic group but from a different generation).
- The unwritten 'rules' relating to non-verbal communication are generally understood within a certain culture but can vary from culture to culture and also from generation to generation. However, it is important to ask or find out individual preferences where possible, as not everyone 'fits in' to these norms. These rules are particularly relevant in the areas of touching, eye contact and the use of personal space. Take the time to understand these for the different cultures you may come across in your professional practice.
- If colleagues and/or patients do not share English as their first language, make sure you give adequate time in communication encounters and obtain feedback to clarify understanding.
- Avoid inappropriate or gratuitous references to a person's culture, etc. For example, "The new patient admitted this morning is a woman by the name of Mary Connolly. She's Irish." By referring to their cultural identity you are implying they are somehow different, so avoid this type of description.

It is common practice in most healthcare settings to use communication tools when caring for patients who do not speak or understand English. In some situations, nurses may rely on family members and friends to communicate with diverse patients. While this may sometimes be useful, it is important to remember that using family, friends and children to communicate is not always effective and may be unethical. Be mindful of your duty to gain consent and of respecting confidentiality. Some cultures have strict rules about sharing health information with children, families or friends, so it cannot be assumed that this is appropriate (Bramhall, 2014; Holland and Hogg, 2010). Employed interpreters should be carefully monitored to ensure communication is effective, and training should be provided to improve this as far as possible. The use of technology is also being increasingly trialled by some institutions, for example through the development of digital communication tools to enhance communication with those patients who need an interpreter when there is none present or available (Silvera-Tawil *et al.*, 2018).

Communicating effectively should be a priority no matter what barriers are perceived. The suggestions below relate to communication episodes where you may be having difficulty with patients who do not speak English. However, they are useful to consider in all communication encounters.

- Book an interpreter. The NHS and care organisations have many services that can be utilised.
- Adopt a calm, welcoming, kind and understanding approach. Remember the patient will be anxious about their language barrier.

■ Use objects and role modelling. For example, show a cup and role model the action of drinking if you want to encourage a patient to increase their fluid intake.

■ Use pictures and simple signs. For example, showing a picture of someone walking with a frame, prior to you helping the patient carry out this activity. Don't underestimate the power of simple drawing; you don't need to be an artist. Hieroglyphics were once the essence of communication and imagery remains a powerful method for imparting and receiving information.

6.3.7 Disability

In addition to differences relating to culture, religion, sexual orientation, age and language, diversity also encompasses the large cohorts of people in society who are physically or learning disabled. People who are blind, partially blind, deaf or partially deaf, and those with autistic spectrum disorders such as autism, Down's syndrome and some mental health conditions, additionally need special attention paid to communicating effectively with them during care delivery. See *Chapter 5* for more information on communicating well with people who need this type of special attention.

6.3.8 Visibility

It is likely that patient groups will consist of varied individuals who may be visible or non-visible minorities (Watson, 2017). Visible diversity encompasses BAME people, older people and people with a physical or certain types of learning disability, such as Down's syndrome.

Refugee migrants from different parts of the world are likely to be visible minorities, although they may also speak English as their second language. Migrants from Europe who may be white and speak English as a second language may still struggle with language barriers. Small groups of migrants, such as some from Polish communities living in rural areas, have stayed within their communities. They may still continue to struggle with communication, even though they are not fully visible (being white) and are not necessarily new migrants to the community (Watson, 2017).

It is important that each person is assessed and treated as an individual rather than on perceptions of how they present themselves and what they look like. This provides the basis for ensuring your communications skills are relevant and sensitive to the needs of individuals and groups that you may encounter as part of your daily practice.

6.3.9 Intersectionality

It is important to remember that individuals may be diverse in more than one of the ways we have described above. Intersectionality is a term that is now increasingly referred to in social sciences research (Clarke and McCall, 2014). Emerging from feminist theorists, it refers to the combination of factors that can contribute to having a negative impact on individual experiences. It could compromise the effective delivery of care and has now become a mainstream discourse in social sciences research relating to oppressive and discriminatory practice. For example, an older woman who is also physically disabled, gay and from a BAME background, may experience the effects of multiple oppressive actions, based on gender, disability, sexual orientation and ethnicity. Some of those actions may be conscious or unconscious, but nonetheless contribute to a discriminatory effect and a strong possibility of negative health outcomes. Unconscious bias will be discussed later in this chapter.

The same is true for older patients from BAME backgrounds, whose first language may not be English, or older patients who are deaf, blind or physically or learning disabled. The intersectional impact of multiple and complex problems can result in making patients very distressed and can severely compromise the communication encounter and delivery of care.

6.4 Communicating with diverse colleagues

It is likely that as a student and when you qualify as a practitioner, you will work with colleagues who are from different backgrounds and cultures. The NHS, as one of the largest employers in Europe, employs a very diverse group of employees locally, nationally and from different parts of the world, in order to meet the needs of service provision on a daily basis. Ensuring that your communication skills are fit for purpose will be an important consideration when you work and study in the healthcare arena. Some useful statistics indicating the diversity of NHS staff are shown in *Figure 6.2*.

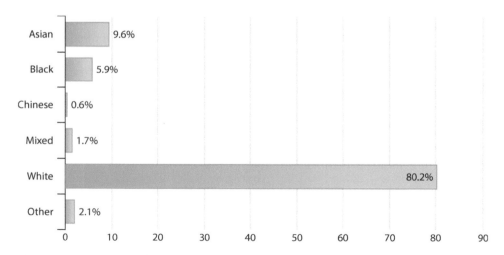

Figure 6.2 *Percentage of NHS staff by ethnicity in England, September 2017–March 2018.*
Source: NHS Digital. Ethnicity Facts and Figures.

ACTIVITY 6.3

What do you think the statistics in *Figure 6.2* show? Were these as you expected?

What other data/information would be useful to search? Think about relevant percentages of ethnicity in varying roles within the NHS. Access the following website for further information: www.ethnicity-facts-figures.service.gov.uk/workforce-and-business/workforce-diversity/nhs-workforce/latest

You can also reach this website by scanning the QR code on the right on your phone.

Developing effective strategies for communication with peers and colleagues is therefore a requirement of every nurse's role. This does not simply apply to colleagues from other cultures, but also to those who may be from a similar culture to yours but have different social or other perspectives. For example, there could be regional differences which may lead to difficulties in understanding speech or behaviours of individuals in the workplace.

ACTIVITY 6.4

Spend ten minutes thinking of an experience where you communicated with:
- A colleague or peer who is from a different part of the UK from you.
- Someone from a different country, whose native language is not English.

What were the factors that helped you to communicate with that person?

What communication aids did you use (give examples)?

What were the barriers that interfered?

How easy/difficult was it to communicate effectively?

You may not have thought about colleagues from regions of the country where accents may be different from yours, given that it is widely recognised that there are regional variations in the use of language in different parts of the UK, even though this may have contributed to slowing down your understanding of what they are saying. Factors that may have helped you could simply be the fact that you share the same ethnicity or culture, or even gender. In any event, paying extra attention to communication patterns in these scenarios should achieve the objective of enabling you to better understand each other and make the day-to-day working relationship much more effective. Individuals who share the same cultural characteristics frequently have episodes of miscommunication, which may be based on a variety of differences, not just from those with different cultural backgrounds. There is simply a requirement to actively engage in understanding the barriers and finding appropriate solutions to overcome them. The important point to note is that addressing the issues is an active process of learning, which applies concepts learned to actual situations being experienced.

Additionally, working with colleagues as well as patients from LGBTQ communities will also require you to show awareness of your style of communication and use of language in order to ensure that it is appropriate and inclusive in different circumstances (Borschman and Marino, 2019). Understanding the issues that may interfere with your communication with different colleagues, some of whom may speak English as a second language and/or may be LGBTQ, is as important as those relating to your patients, given the diversity in the NHS workforce (Rein, 2016). Interprofessional and intercultural communication with doctors and other colleagues whose native language is not English could have safety implications if due care is not taken. Workplace staffing issues of chronic shortages and rapid staff turnover make it imperative that good practice is fostered at all levels.

6.4.1 Unconscious bias

Communicating in any setting is always influenced by varying factors, of which the participants may or may not be aware. These factors are based on perceptions, stereotypes and/or personal and past experiences, and have the capacity to influence the communication episode either positively or negatively. Referred to as unconscious or implicit bias, this can occur when an individual's background, experiences and other sociocultural context unknowingly interferes with decision-making. This may, however, have negative outcomes when those decisions affect other individuals or groups (Equality Challenge Unit, 2018).

The term originates from the discipline of psychology (Flarman, 2016), and supports the view that everyone is biased simply because of the way our brains are structured to receive and respond to external stimuli. An individual has to first become aware of their biases before they are able to positively address them. They can then begin to take decisive actions to reverse negative outcomes that may affect other people (Equality Challenge Unit, 2018). Admitting to bias is difficult, because it could conjure up a state of possible discomfort or denial, as it forces individuals to move out of their comfort zones.

While unconscious bias may appear to be a fairly straightforward issue, in terms of admission of bias, the term is still contested by some and seen as one more way of distracting from the real issue of discrimination, which is pervasive in all social structures. When manifested in daily actions, it is suggested that people can be affected by a range of social and physical stimuli, including but not limited to dress, accent, a person's physical appearance, ethnicity, skin colour, sexual orientation or other known diverse factors about the individual or their cohort (Borschman and Marino, 2019). Behaviours may be manifested by actions that may be covert, or hidden, such as regular daily micro-aggressive actions that are minor but gradually add up to make people at whom the actions are directed feel that they do not belong or are not appreciated. Irish *et al.*'s (2018) research suggests LGBTQ people particularly identify this as having a negative impact on their lives, seeing this as a major trigger of their depression and suicidal thoughts.

It is well documented that such stereotypical assumptions are not uncommon in society (Watson, 2017), and even though many initiatives have been made by policy-makers and public and private employers to address the issues, they are still pervasive (RCN, 2012).

Unconscious bias training seeks to provide further support by enabling individuals to question their actions and address gaps in personal beliefs. The overall aim is to encourage everyone to consider how they respond to difference in the workplace and to take action that will change their own perceptions and/or challenge the perceptions of others. This ensures the recognition that understanding and responding to diversity and difference in all settings, but especially in public sector environments such as the NHS work environments, is an important contributor to good practice, and must become everyone's business (RCN, 2012).

ACTIVITY 6.5

Now that we have established we are all biased, this activity should help you to identify some of your biases. But first, think about the following question:

Would you agree that you have some biases?

Spend a few minutes thinking about some that you are prepared to admit to, or that you are definitely aware of.

To help you, here is an initial list of possibilities, but it is not exhaustive. Can you think of others?
1.   People who are very short
2.   People who are very obese
3.   People who are vegans
4.   People from a different culture
5.   People from a different country
6.   People of a different religion
7.   People who are gay

How many others did you think of?

As an example, while you may not have chosen people who are very fat, it is important for you to be aware that those who are obese in our 'body conscious' society often feel stigmatised and that they do not fit in. There is an increasing social emphasis on diet and healthy eating, so we may presume that someone who is obese, eats a poor diet and doesn't exercise may be lazy. Additionally, we are exposed to the social media celebrity culture, which expects women to have model-like silhouettes, usually very thin, with long legs. There is now a small shift in awareness and encouragement to enable women to be comfortable with their own bodies regardless of their size. However, because of the likely impact on health and wellbeing, and in the light of the current increase in diseases such as diabetes, this is still a very sensitive area which makes individuals very self-conscious. Communication with awareness, empathy and encouragement is paramount to reduce all feelings of guilt and self-hatred.

Jennifer Mieres is a cardiologist and medical director in the USA. She has proposed five ways to mitigate unconscious bias, which are listed below and should be considered carefully when engaging in communication activity (Mieres, 2005):

- Recognise and accept that everyone (including your patients) has biases. Biases, when challenged, may not be based on rational reality but on previous emotional or social experiences.
- Shine a light on yourself. Develop a capacity to learn about yourself, as the more you observe yourself, the more aware you will become of how you behave towards others.
- Practise constructive uncertainty. This means challenging preconceived ideas you have about yourself and others. Don't always think you are certain; check your assumptions. Try asking questions from a non-judgemental stance and consult others.
- Explore awkwardness and discomfort. It is OK to feel awkward in situations you are not used to. Being outside your comfort zone can be a great opportunity for learning. This can help you to then reflect on situations where you can subsequently challenge your own and others' behaviours in the future, when you feel more confident.
- Learn about people. Engage with people you would not normally socialise with. Consciously learn about other cultures to dispel myths and assumptions about stereotypes. Ask for feedback from others about your own behaviours.

6.4.2 Addressing discriminatory practice

The NHS workplace remains a diverse place in which to work, and provides opportunities to experience a richness of cultures, people and populations. Once you have developed your own self-awareness, you may wish to become a Diversity Champion for the Royal College of Nursing (RCN, 2012). This is a position that recognises your increasing awareness of the importance of diversity in all clinical environments, and of your commitment to do something positive about it through actively making decisions fairly, challenging unfairness and/or promoting an environment of inclusiveness in your workplace. A diversity champion seeks to ensure that NHS workplaces become more responsive to diverse patient and staff needs and strives to keep everyone aware of their responsibilities to contribute to positive care outcomes at all times.

When considering your workplace responses to patients, carers and their families, or to your colleagues, it is important to use your awareness of the issues that could interfere with your communication skills. Once you have ensured an understanding of your actions, you should have clear strategies to achieve a successful outcome. Before you undertake any kind of communication that could potentially be difficult, remember to think about the specific issues that could make it even more problematic (Hull, 2016; James and Szeman, 2010). If necessary, seek help before you begin, and as far as possible, make sure it is identified as part of your assessment, planning and care delivery action plan for that particular patient. These issues could include, for example, language or other barriers that may interfere, such as cultural differences in the perception of personal or intimate care from those of the opposite sex in a care delivery episode, or understanding issues relating to therapeutic touch, eye contact and non-verbal communication.

It is useful to remember, as stated earlier, that some people who are very ill and distressed physically, emotionally and/or mentally, may not be able to express themselves clearly in what to them could be a strange, bustling and noisy ward or clinic. You have a responsibility to be sensitive to the requirements of all patients, whatever their diverse situation may be, and devise a planned response to ensure a successful care delivery outcome. It is good practice to ensure that your colleagues and peers are given feedback on any episode of difficult communication with any diverse group through written and verbal reports. Critically reflecting on these encounters and learning from them will help you as you develop and build on your experiences in the health workplace.

Below is a checklist of other areas to consider:
1. Make sure that you are clear about the preferred ways of communicating that any particular individual prefers.
2. Ensure that the setting is optimal and one in which the individual will be comfortable.
3. If this is someone with whom you are communicating for the first time, pay attention to the way they are receiving information from you, as this will be useful for any future communication episodes.
4. Determine the amount of information that any individual can process, and whether there is a case to only share on a need to know basis, with reasons for your decisions, perhaps based on the patient's or carer's personal circumstances.
5. Aim to reach an agreeable stage of giving information, so that individuals do not feel left out or spoken down to.
6. Make sure that you are clear about the member of staff who is best placed to provide information or receive feedback.
7. Be clear about the best ways of giving or receiving information for each individual episode.

ACTIVITY 6.6

Find who the Diversity Lead or Champions are in your placement area or NHS Trust.

Arrange to speak with them, either electronically or in person where possible.

Find out about their role and share your findings with your peers/colleagues in practice.

Do you feel the role is fit for purpose? Would you become one? Why or why not?

The case study below is based on real examples from practice, with all names changed for confidentiality purposes (NMC, 2018). It gives you an opportunity to explore possible clinical scenarios.

CASE STUDY

You are a staff nurse working a night duty shift on a surgical ward. Along with the ward sister, you have a second-year student, Lindsay, John, a first-year student nurse, and David, a healthcare assistant (HCA). John was a former HCA and is very confident, but this is his first night duty shift. Under your supervision, he is looking after a male Asian Sikh patient, Baljit, 35 years old, who has a mild learning disability and is an insulin-dependent diabetic. He had been stabilised following his operation, is self-caring and self-medicating with his insulin, and is due to go home the next day. Lindsay, your second-year student, is providing care for a patient on the female side of the ward, also under your supervision. The patient, Alia Mertha, is 68 years old, had a cholecystectomy operation late that evening and requires post-operative care during the night. Alia is originally from Romania and speaks a little English.

Dr Mensa, a migrant doctor from Lithuania, is the on-call surgical officer on night duty. During the night, Alia Mertha is very restless, demanding and noisy. In the morning the doctor arrives on the ward to check that everything is satisfactory before he goes off duty. He asks Lindsay for an update on Mrs Mertha's progress during the night. Lindsay casually says to the doctor, "Alia is a pain in the neck". Doctor Mensa gets agitated and asks why no one had informed him during the night that his patient had a pain in the neck. There is shock and surprise that the doctor has misunderstood the communication, and Lindsay laughs and tries to reassure the doctor that the patient did not have a pain in the neck but was very demanding throughout the night. The doctor appears puzzled and confused and comes to the ward office to ask you for further explanation.

- What are the cross-cultural issues in this episode of communication?
- As the staff nurse supervising the student that night, how would you respond to the doctor?
- What would be your feedback to Lindsay?
- How could this be prevented in the future?

During the early part of your night shift, Baljit's only sister Sukhi visited the ward requesting to see her brother. She had travelled from out of town to make sure his discharge arrangements were satisfactory for the next day. Although visiting hours were over, John took Sukhi into the male bay to see her brother straight away, as he didn't want to be accused of being racially discriminatory. John and Sukhi (without including Baljit) had a discussion about his discharge arrangements. She told John she had come down to be there for her brother as he was not very bright, and that he would need support because he could not communicate very well. She would be staying at a local hotel that night and would return the next day to take him home to his flat.

You returned to duty the next night and were told by the handover team that Baljit's key worker had telephoned just after you left that morning, saying that Baljit had contacted him very upset and distressed. Baljit had complained that he had not been consulted about his sister's plans and that John and Sukhi spoke about him in the room as if he wasn't there. Baljit had a girlfriend with whom he was living, who his sister did not know about because she hadn't seen him for many years. Arrangements had been made for Baljit to be picked up by his key worker that morning and taken to his flat, where his girlfriend would be waiting for him. Neither John nor Sukhi knew about Baljit's arrangements as they did not ask him. The handover had simply said that Baljit would be discharged in the morning.

- What are the issues of concern in this scenario?
- What actions may be taken to achieve a positive patient experience?
- Going forward, what would you do to ensure this does not happen to another patient?

Some areas you may wish to consider include:

Expectations relating to use of language and everyday English colloquialisms/terminology.

Likely patient safety implications.

Unconscious bias.

Implicit assumptions of disability, ethnicity and care participation/inclusion.

Summary

Assumptions about any patient who is different can be unconscious and hence discriminatory. Every patient should be included in any discussion about their care. Communicating effectively in diverse situations is a challenging but required skill for delivering culturally competent care to all patients, service users and families. Complex and challenging communication skills can be developed by showing awareness and commitment to improving care delivery to everyone. Colloquial terminology should be avoided, given the risks and safety implications for intercultural and interprofessional misunderstandings and the likely impact on patient experience.

KEY LEARNING POINTS

Six key points to take away from *Chapter 6*:
- ☑ Communication in diversity is enhanced by a clearer understanding of globalised and diverse localised social contexts and their impact on patients as individuals.
- ☑ Getting diverse communication right has the benefit of enhancing patient satisfaction and improving patient safety, while ensuring that all caregivers, including staff, and families are satisfied with their contribution to the process.
- ☑ It is not enough to simply learn about cultural differences. Nurses should recognise the intersectional impact of ethnicity, gender, class and sexual orientation and their potential to contribute to multiple oppressive actions and health disparities.
- ☑ Nurses can engage directly with individual patients about their specific healthcare needs so that the risk of stereotyping can be reduced. This can be done using relevant helpful tools of communication to assist this process.
- ☑ Challenges to communication within a diverse context can be overcome with appropriate assessment, design and planning prior to implementing care. This should be identified as an integral aspect of the assessment process, and properly evaluated following an episode of care.
- ☑ Engaging with, or becoming, a Diversity Champion is one aspect of good practice that can be shared with other colleagues to enable a continued improved satisfaction experience for all patients and staff.

FURTHER READING

Anderson, K.J. (2010) *Benign Bigotry: the psychology of subtle prejudice.* Cambridge University Press.

Hynes, G.E. (2015) *Get Along, Get It Done, Get Ahead: interpersonal communication in the diverse workplace.* Business Expert Press.

Phillips, T. and Phillips, M. (1999) *Windrush: the irresistible rise of multi-racial Britain.* Harper Collins.

REFERENCES

Borschman, R. and Marino, J. (2019) Sexual identity and mental health in young people: an opportunity to reduce health inequity. *The Lancet: Child & Adolescent Health,* **3(2)**: 57–9.

Bramhall, E. (2014) Effective communication skills in nursing practice. *Nursing Standard,* **29(14)**: 53–9.

Clarke, A.Y. and McCall, L. (2014) Intersectionality and social explanation in social science research. *Du Bois Review,* **10(2)**: 349–63.

Crisp, R.J. and Meleady, R. (2012) Adapting to a multicultural future. *Science,* **336(6083)**: 853–5.

Equality and Human Rights Commission (2013) Equality Act 2010: guidance. Available at: www.gov.uk/guidance/equality-act-2010-guidance (accessed 19 July 2019).

Equality Challenge Unit (ECU)/Advance HE (2018) *Unconscious Bias.* London ECU/Advance HE.

Flarman, S.E. (2016) Unconscious bias: when good intentions aren't enough. *Educational Leadership,* **74(3)**: 10–15.

Holland, K. and Hogg, C. (2010) *Cultural Awareness in Health and Social Care.* Edward Arnold.

Hull, M. (2016) Medical language proficiency: a discussion of interprofessional language competencies and potential patient risk. *International Journal of Nursing Studies,* **54**: 158–72.

Irish, M., Solmi, F., Mars, B. *et al.* (2018) Depression and self-harm from adolescence to young adulthood in sexual minorities compared with heterosexuals in the UK: a population-based cohort study. *The Lancet: Child & Adolescent Health,* **3(2)**: 91–8.

James, P. and Szeman, I. (2010) *Globalization and Culture, Vol. 3. Global-local consumption*. Sage.

Mieres, J. (2005) Gender- and race-based differences in CVD. *Journal of Family Practice*, Supplement 3.

New South Wales Department of Education and Training (2009) *Belonging: Calendar for Cultural Diversity 2010: information for teachers and students*. Department of Education and Training, Multicultural Programs Unit.

Nursing and Midwifery Council (2018) *The Code: professional standards of practice and behaviour for nurses, midwives and nursing associates*. NMC. Available at: www.nmc.org.uk/globalassets/sitedocuments/nmc-publications/nmc-code.pdf (accessed 19 July 2019).

Office for National Statistics (2012) *2011 Census: Key Statistics for England and Wales, March 2011*. Available at: www.ons.gov.uk/peoplepopulationand community/populationandmigration/populationestimates/bulletins/2011 censuskeystatisticsforenglandandwales/2012-12-11 (accessed 19 July 2019).

Rein, R. (2016) *Meaning in Action. Outline of an Integral Meaning of Culture*. Polity Press.

Royal College of Nursing (2012) *Diversity Champions*. RCN.

Silvera-Tawil, D., Pocock, C., Bradford, D. *et al.* (2018) CALD Assist–Nursing: improving communication in the absence of interpreters. *Journal of Clinical Nursing*, **27(21–22)**: 4168–78.

Sleek, S. (2018) The bias beneath two decades of measuring implicit associations. *APS Observer*, **31(2)**: 11–14.

Watson, N.A. (2017) *"Here to stay…so… deal with it…": experiences and perceptions of Black British African Caribbean people about nursing careers*. Lambeth Academic Publishing.

Chapter 7

Communication skills for teamworking

Kay Norman

LEARNING OUTCOMES

By the end of this chapter you should be able to:

7.1 Be aware of the various approaches available to promote effective communication in teams

7.2 Reflect on how you and other individuals negotiate care as part of a team and within an organisation

7.3 Understand the importance of collaborative working in communicating the planning and delivery of nursing care

7.4 Explain effective communication approaches in a supervisory relationship.

7.1 Introduction

Teamworking is fundamental to successful nursing care. Even as a lone worker in a community or clinic setting, there will be members of staff from a range of backgrounds who may be involved in some way to ensure patient care is appropriate, effective, efficient and meets all required needs.

You will appreciate teams can consist of few or many participants and have a variety of remits. For example, assigning teams as part of a project initiative to set up a new walk-in emergency service requires people with specific skills such as clinicians (medical staff, nurses, paramedics, midwives), finance staff, administrative/management staff, estates personnel. A 'care' team that focuses on a particular area of nursing, such as community care, may involve a team with a specific skill mix such as a specialist practitioner, staff nurses and healthcare assistants (HCAs). However, they will also liaise with the wider healthcare team such as social workers, GPs, physiotherapists, occupational therapists, voluntary sector agencies and hospital discharge planners. Therefore in today's healthcare systems, 'teams' need to be collaborative and not tribalistic, communicating and working with others to enable a consistent approach for the patient, community and service.

This chapter will explore possible influencing factors that can affect team communication, including strategies that can be employed to address potential areas of conflict.

7.2 Strengths-based approaches

Strengths-based approaches to teamwork have been developed within the business sector over many years. This approach suggests that individuals should acknowledge and appreciate their strengths (skills, knowledge and talent) to offer these in a team environment. Rather than trying to fix or improve perceived or real 'weaknesses', drawing on strengths will improve performance (Curtis and Cullen, 2017). Clearly communicating and reiterating your strengths to others will help identify your place within a team and also clarify expectations. One of the benefits of teamwork is the individual strengths of its members. This is not to say you cannot work to improve your limitations; however, research has suggested that teams are not only more efficient, but also happier using this approach. So how do you communicate your strengths to others?

From *Figure 7.1*, list your talent, skills and knowledge. Add to this by asking colleagues, mentors, peers, friends, family and any significant others for their thoughts also.

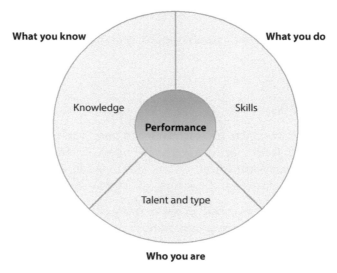

Figure 7.1 *Performance wheel.*

It may surprise you to discover what others perceive your strengths to be. Often, we can work with colleagues on a daily basis without realising what their particular strengths are, unless they are allowed to express them and are encouraged to use them. By using the above activity with your team, everyone can begin to appreciate how each individual can be more effective, better utilised, and feel valued in their role. This team could include your fellow students, a small nursing team allocated to a specific group of patients, a larger ward team involving members of the MDT, a community nursing team, or a general practice team involving nurses/ HCAs, and medical and administration staff.

- Ask the team leader if this activity can be explored at the next available meeting.
- Explain the purpose prior to the meeting taking place.
- Ensure there is an opportunity for individuals to ask questions to ensure they understand the benefits of the activity.
- Stipulate a time limit for completing the activity, discussing and disseminating the outcomes.

It is this open, sharing approach, acknowledging an individual's strengths, which can form a good basis on which to grow an effective team. However, an additional desired outcome of adopting strengths-based practice is team resilience. The starting point to remember is 'what is right' with people, what the positive attributes of that person are. As a student nurse, you will develop and build individual resilience throughout your learning journey in order to plan and practise safe nursing care. Resilience can be defined as "the ability of an individual to cope with and adapt positively to adverse circumstances" (Hunter and Warren, 2013). Nevertheless, team resilience can also be built in supporting each other through periods of change and uncertainty, thereby increasing retention of staff. Teams are mini-organisations. As you move forward to a registered nurse, you don't need to be everyone's friend but you do need to encourage, instil a sense of self-worth, and facilitate a sense of belonging in your team and co-workers. You are all in this together!

According to Hammond (2010), the mindset of a resilient person has the following characteristics – they:

- feel special and appreciated – they have a strong sense of hope and optimism
- view life as a dynamic journey that involves them writing the next chapters – by how they perceive themselves and who they invite on the trip
- have learned to set realistic goals and expectations for themselves
- rely on productive coping strategies that are growth-fostering rather than self-defeating
- view obstacles as challenges to confront – not avoid
- are aware of their weaknesses and vulnerabilities, but purposefully build on strengths
- have strong self-esteem and sense of competence
- have effective interpersonal skills and can seek out assistance and nurturance from others (formal and informal relationships)
- know what they can and cannot control in their lives
- have a strong understanding of the need to give back – they support others in their journey.

As individuals relate to this mindset, team resilience will be fostered.

ACTIVITY 7.1

Think about a recent practice experience. Reflect on the individuals that made up the 'team'. How did they support each other? What were the challenges and how were these managed? How did they communicate with others as a whole team?

From this experience, what strategies would you use to communicate with your team to build team resilience?

Some areas you might consider:

- Tools and exercises available. There are numerous online resources to plan activities (see Further reading).

- Goals are communicated effectively – check understanding and a shared ownership.

- Clarity of team purpose.

- Interdependence – appreciate that each individual's contribution is needed for a successful outcome.

- Empowerment – individuals feel they are valuable in achieving the desired outcome and have influence on decisions.

- Willingness of individuals to engage in a unified objective.

- Active listening.

- Recognition of different communication styles in the team.

- Valuing diverse ideas.

- Scheduled focused meetings to recap, assess progress/challenges and agree actions to move forward.

7.3 Negotiation strategies

The importance of team dynamics cannot be underestimated; how team members engage with each other to plan and deliver care will make a difference to how effectively the team functions. A designated 'lead' can steer the team in terms of how they work together, but all members of the team have a role to play. Belbin (2010) continues to influence theories of teamwork based on initial work related to behaviours, identifying nine roles seen within teams. Knowing your team members and their role within the team will help you plan and prepare negotiating strategies. For example, you may need to negotiate an off-duty rota, work out how best to implement an audit process, negotiate changing roles and responsibilities, identify resources for further education and training, or develop new ways of working within the service/department to ensure efficient and effective care.

Review the nine behaviours shown in *Table 7.1*. Do they resonate with teams you have previously worked with? Not all roles will be present in each team and some individuals may display more than one role. Can you identify *your* current role within a team?

Table 7.1 *Behaviours identified in teams*

Role	Strengths	Limitations	However….
Resource investigator Finds ideas to bring back to the team	Outgoing, enthusiastic, explores opportunities and develops contacts	Can be over-optimistic. Can lose interest after initial enthusiasm	They might forget to follow up a lead
Teamworker Helps the team to gel	Cooperative, perceptive and diplomatic. Listens and averts friction	Can be indecisive in crunch situations and tends to avoid confrontation	They might be hesitant to make unpopular decisions
Coordinator Focused on team objectives. Delegates to get the work done	Mature, confident, identifies talent. Clarifies goals	Can be seen as manipulative and might offload their own share of the work	May over-delegate, leaving themselves little work to do
Plant Good at solving problems creatively	Creative, imaginative, free-thinking, generates ideas, and solves difficult problems	Might ignore incidentals, may be too preoccupied to communicate effectively	They could be absent-minded or forgetful
Monitor evaluator Makes impartial judgements, weighs up options	Logical, strategic and discerning. Sees all options and judges accurately	Sometimes lacks drive and ability to inspire others, can be overly critical	They could be slow to come to decisions
Specialist Brings in-depth knowledge/skills to the team	Single-minded, self-starting and dedicated. They provide specialist knowledge and skills	Tends to contribute on a narrow front and can dwell on the technicalities	They may overload you with information
Shaper Provides drive to ensure the team keeps focused and doesn't lose momentum	Challenging, dynamic, thrives on pressure. Has the drive and courage to overcome obstacles	Can be prone to provocation and may sometimes hurt people's feelings	They could risk becoming aggressive and bad-humoured in their attempts to get things done

(continued)

Table 7.1 *(continued)*

Role	Strengths	Limitations	However….
Implementer Plans a workable strategy to carry it out as efficiently as possible	Practical, reliable, efficient. Turns ideas into actions and organises work that needs to be done	Can be a bit inflexible and slow to respond to new possibilities.	They may be slow to relinquish their plans in favour of positive changes.
Completer/finisher Used at end of tasks to scrutinise for errors, high standard of quality control.	Painstaking, conscientious, anxious. Searches out errors. Polishes and perfects.	Can be inclined to worry unduly, and reluctant to delegate.	They could be accused of taking their perfectionism to extremes.

Source: Belbin (2010): www.belbin.com/about/belbin-team-roles

In order to negotiate successful outcomes within a team, it is important to prepare. Know your team and the players involved as this will provide valuable information on who you feel would be best suited to a particular role, who may be difficult to convince, who will help to inspire others, who will provide honest feedback. Also think about your own position – how will people view your role in this negotiation? Communicating clearly with all team members to ensure understanding is key to being a successful negotiator. Think about following up discussions with a draft written summary, which needs to be agreed by all members for clarity and accuracy. Sometimes what you think was said and agreed in a meeting may not be interpreted in the same way by everyone. Consider those members of the team who could not attend the face-to-face discussion. If possible, arrange a face-to-face follow-up or Skype call to see their reaction and body language. The key points when preparing for negotiating are:

- Know your team.
- Send out preparation material. In addition to a scheduled agenda, this could be reading a report, completing an activity, asking for contributions on a particular theme.
- Be clear about what you hope to achieve and be realistic. Use SMART objectives.
- Be prepared for conflict.
- Consider a variety of options and possible consequences.
- Think about possible solutions and compromises.
- Plan for follow-up.
- Practise being persuasive. Help people to make a decision.

In order to negotiate successful outcomes, people need to feel you have their best interests and those of the patients in mind. When considering a request for action, consider all responses. The aim should always be a commitment to act, which is the first step to achieving the end goal. List small achievable objectives that can be negotiated.

Forsyth (2009) suggests that there are two key factors to remember when negotiating in a team: how you project yourself (confidence, credibility) and how you demonstrate empathy in the ability to see things from their viewpoint.

Here are some tips that will help you in negotiating:

- Be positive and identify the one thing that you need to have agreement on and those that you can take forward to the next meeting. Be prepared for those points that may become loss leaders.
- Relay your suggestions and underpinning evidence base.
- Be confident to move the discussion forward and try to keep to the time schedule for each agenda item.
- Be mindful to summarise each agreed action point.
- Schedule time to hear viewpoints and acknowledge contributions. Use effective verbal and non-verbal communication skills to portray empathy (see *Chapter 1*).

Everyone needs to feel they are satisfied to some extent with the outcome, even if they don't necessarily agree with it. For example, you are negotiating a change in shift patterns to deal with winter pressures on an acute medical ward. Many do not agree with working a 24-hour shift pattern, although they can understand the reasons due to shortage of staff. In order to negotiate this change, it has been agreed that the change in shift pattern will only be for one month to ease pressures, and not a permanent change.

ACTIVITY 7.2

Reflect on a previous episode where your team has needed to negotiate a change. How was this managed? Analyse the roles people adopted. Was this planned effectively and how were actions implemented. Did this result in a win–win outcome where all members felt some sense of satisfaction? List the actions you would do differently and what you feel worked well.

7.4 Collaborative working

Collaborative working has taken on different meanings depending on the people and organisations involved. You may also hear this term used interchangeably with partnership working and integrated working/care. Here are some definitions which you should consider when applying this term to your everyday practice:

- "The act of two or more people working together for a particular purpose." *Cambridge Business English Dictionary*
- "A whole systems perspective, not just two organisations working together. It is about encompassing agencies and departments and the relationships between them and the service user/citizen." *(Miles and Trott, 2011)*
- "Collaborative working involves working together through sharing ideas to provide solutions, a strong sense of purpose and equal participation." https://study.com/academy/lesson/what-is-collaboration-in-the-workplace-definition-benefits-examples.html
- "Being committed to working and engaging constructively with internal and external stakeholders." *Institute for Innovation and Improvement*

The NMC *Code* states that "you must work in partnership with people to make sure you deliver care effectively" (NMC, 2018, p. 5). Collaborative working may seem common sense in teamworking and much collaboration literature suggests that it is, in essence, taking teamwork further. However, as lessons from history can illustrate, the ability to apply collaborative communication in situations where we feel threatened can prove difficult. Groups can become tribalistic and feel safer when surrounded by people with like-minded values and beliefs. However, in complex and diverse societies such as our own, the ability to communicate collaboratively with those who differ from ourselves is essential.

Numerous studies have suggested that collaborative communication between all personnel involved with patient care improves patient safety and outcomes. It has also been suggested that this promotes consistency of treatment delivery, and reduces the risk of errors in patient care. Nevertheless, many disciplines and groups continue to operate as separate healthcare providers with very few episodes of collaborative discussion (Cornell and Townsend-Gervis, 2014; Lancaster *et al.*, 2015; Radtke, 2013).

Think for a minute about the range of personnel you know who have input to patient care. This might include a variety of nurses, medical staff, social workers, allied health professionals, specialist services, paramedics and voluntary agencies. Do you know much about their specific roles? Do you communicate with them on a regular basis? Literature suggests that in order to collaborate effectively, each 'player' needs to understand the other's role, expertise and how they can contribute to the improvement of a situation or episode of care (Karam *et al.*, 2018). *Table 7.2* identifies some requirements needed to promote positive collaborative communication and also possible barriers. Can you think of any others? When you think about your own team and others you work with, do you recognise some of the positive factors and barriers?

Table 7.2 *Promoters and barriers to collaborative communication*

Factors promoting positive collaborative communication	Barriers to successful collaborative communication
Understanding of each others' roles and responsibilities	Personal values and expectations
Patient-centredness	Historical professional rivalries
Organisational positivity (NHS Trust)	Perceptions of hierarchy
Open and honest interactions	Differences in language or terminology
Formal and informal meetings	Status/unequal power/not feeling opinions are valued
Regular opportunities to discuss issues	No confidence in others

(continued)

Table 7.2 (continued)

Factors promoting positive collaborative communication	Barriers to successful collaborative communication
Shared power	Gender
Interdependence	Differences in regulations
	Disruptive behaviour/unwillingness
	Responsibility for decision-making

ACTIVITY 7.3

Consider a recent patient you have been involved with as the centre of collaborative working. How many health professionals and other agencies are involved in their care? List your understanding and perceptions of each role and how you feel collaborative communication is meeting the patient's needs. Take some time to research each role and talk to each healthcare professional/agency personnel about their specific expertise. Has it changed your perception?

Drawing on the communication strategies discussed so far in this book, map how you would plan effective collaborative communication to ensure the patient's needs are met efficiently and consistently.

Bhatt and Mitchell (2015) suggest that both positive and negative factors need to be discussed within collaborative groups to encourage an open honest dialogue, promoting understanding of each others' role and perspectives. As this can take time, in particular to break down barriers of professional rivalries and hierarchy, all members must demonstrate a willingness to accept others from the outset. To this end, the culture of an organisation will ultimately affect how all staff develop team and collaborative communication skills as an absolute requisite for providing safe, high-quality care.

The King's Fund has produced a toolkit for collaborative teamworking which comprises a seven-step process that staff can work through (King's Fund, 2016). Although it mainly focuses on clinical staff working with finance organisations, the principles apply to all interprofessional working:

- Get the right support
- Invite the right people
- Find out what people think
- Prepare for the session
- Get people talking
- Keep going, make changes, reflect again
- Support each other.

Collaborative communication is a team effort and requires support from all parts of the organisations involved, including chief executives to lead and promote this within a culture of quality. However, all organisations are made up of individuals so we all have a part to play in ensuring this remains a consistent and ongoing process.

7.5 Organisational culture

The Francis Report (2013) identified organisational culture as one of the underpinning areas for reform following the failings in care at Mid Staffordshire NHS Foundation Trust. Organisational culture is again a concept with many definitions; however, the common themes include shared values and norms, repeated behaviours which new staff are socialised into, and 'the way things are done here' (Dixon-Woods *et al.*, 2014). The importance of effective leadership in ensuring positive, innovative and caring organisational cultures cannot be underestimated. However, if staff feel unsupported, not appreciated, have inadequate resources, don't feel listened to and perceive poor leadership, care quality and safety will be threatened.

Organisational culture is made up of many elements and results from individual and team decisions over periods of time. Processes, systems, values and 'norms' emerge that can result in a positive or toxic environment. The context can influence people's choice of behaviour and conformity to group behaviours. A result of a toxic environment can be 'good' people who are influenced to do 'poor' things to fit in with the team/organisation norm, or collude with behaviours that are supported by the boundaries of a corrosive environment. Building individual and organisational capability starts from the self and builds outwards, as seen in the 'building and strengthening leadership' model in *Figure 7.2* (NHS England, 2014). The model also demonstrates that conversely, when diagnosing issues at an organisational level, the start point should be the outside (environment) level working inwards. Each layer can be used to help diagnose and explain behaviours and choices to see where breakdown has occurred.

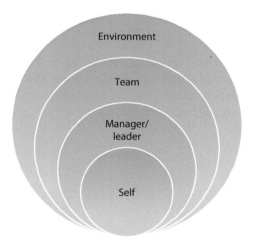

Figure 7.2 *Building and strengthening leadership (NHS England, 2014).*

The NHS Leadership Academy (2017) suggests that developing a positive organisational culture "is about leading change, service improvement initiatives, engaging and motivating staff, developing their talents and improving potential of staff. Great organisational development is about understanding context and culture, taking a systems approach and enabling NHS staff to design and deliver great patient care".

'Engaging the team' is one of the nine dimensions of the Leadership Healthcare Model and relates to all those who have a leadership responsibility, from a one-to-one consultation episode to those leading a large organisation. The way teams perform and react will ultimately affect the organisational culture.

Below are examples of strategies for creating positive cultures. This chapter does not attempt to discuss leadership theory and approaches in depth; however, organisational culture improvement has communication at its core and therefore needs to be included and considered here. As leadership is now seen as 'everyone's business', as a student nurse you will be leading episodes of care, experience professional socialisation into organisations and will lead teams, initiatives and improvements for patient benefit in due course.

Leaders should (West *et al.*, 2011):
- continually reinforce an inspiring vision of the work of their organisations
- promote staff health and wellbeing
- listen to staff and encourage them to be involved in decision-making, problem-solving and innovation at all levels
- provide staff with helpful feedback on how they are doing and celebrate good performance
- take effective, supportive action to address system problems and other challenges when improvement is needed
- develop and model excellent teamwork
- make sure that staff feel safe, supported, respected and valued at work.

However, organisations should communicate with all staff and patients using a variety of ways and multiple strategies to avoid missing particular viewpoints and groups. Dixon-Woods *et al.* (2014) also suggest that self-assessment should be incorporated to evaluate local cultures and behaviours, not just relying on mandated measures. Links are evident where staff feel happy and positive in their workplace, as this results in wellbeing of patients, with staff engagement being a key predictor across a range of NHS outcomes.

As you make the transition from student to registered nurse, your leadership role will continue to develop so it is important to access the variety of sources and literature available on leadership styles and models to have a deeper understanding of your strengths and limitations, areas where you can improve and develop, and identify a suitable role model/mentor. You will find some useful resources in the Further reading section at the end of this chapter.

ACTIVITY 7.4

Do you feel engaged and involved in some way (no matter how small) in the organisational decision-making and planning of care improvements? How do you feel you currently contribute to the organisational culture? Think about how you can meaningfully contribute in the future. What communication strategies would you employ?

You may find it helpful to access the leadership academy model and answer the questions relating to 'engaging the team' dimension as a starting point. Either visit the website below or scan the QR code on the right:

www.leadershipacademy.nhs.uk/resources/healthcare-leadership-model/nine-leadership-dimensions/engaging-the-team/

In the NHS report *Building and Strengthening Leadership: leading with compassion* (NHS England, 2014), compassionate leadership is seen to commence with the individual values and beliefs, although will be affected by the organisational culture of the workplace. It has been widely suggested that compassionate care for patients will be more likely if the individual giving the care feels they are also treated with compassion by their employers. High levels of positive emotion are needed at work to create a culture of compassion.

So how can you, as a future leader of a team, help to encourage a culture of positivity and compassion? NHS England's (2014) action recommendations for leaders and managers in how to engage and develop their teams to promote a compassionate culture are:

- **Get to know your team individually**. Make time for one-to-one discussions. Be honest and encourage dialogue to ascertain what motivates them, what you can do more/less of to motivate them. Ask about their development plans and career progression outcomes.
- **Build a plan to close the engagement gap**.
- Know them (see above).
- Grow them. This will promote a shared vision for their future in the organisation.
- Inspire them. Help them make an emotional connection to their work, with the organisation, with the team. Their skills and interests can inspire others and this contributes to the organisation vision, and generates excitement within the team.
- Involve them. Allow individuals to be creative. An organisation needs to learn daily from its employees and allow discretion in their work.
- Reward them. Find new ways to show appreciation (pay rises will not be available so don't promise rewards that cannot be substantiated). Recognise good work, know if this should be done privately or publicly depending on the individual. Access development opportunities, secondments, coaching. Consider other roles to 'stretch', mentoring.
- **Make strategy and targets meaningful**. When discussing appraisal performance reviews, make the links between personal objectives and organisational goals.
- Be compelling in explaining 'why are we doing this'.

- **Notice the signs and respond.**
- Be aware of changes in behaviours and habits (examples could include being late for shifts, showing weight change, not going to breaks, being more dependent on caffeine, having a change in appearance and/or mood). Use these as a clear sign they need support in ways to re-balance. Know and provide access to available support mechanisms such as counselling services, and think through alternative behaviours.

7.6 Dealing with team conflict

Diverse teams are essential in our current society. They add a wealth of knowledge, skills and cultural understanding to address community and patient needs, in addition to having a voice to represent diversity in decision-making. However, building diverse teams can be difficult. Encouraging collegiality in teams with different backgrounds, language, culture, views and preferences can be challenging. This can lead to mistrust, anxiety and team conflict unless addressed and resolved. This is reflected in Lencioni's (2009) five dysfunctions of a team, as shown in the model in *Table 7.3*, which can be a starting point for action and discussion within your team.

Table 7.3 *The five dysfunctions of a team (Lencioni, 2009)*

Inattention to results	The pursuit of individual goals and personal status erodes the focus on collective success
Avoidance of accountability	The need to avoid interpersonal discomfort prevents team members from holding one another accountable
Lack of commitment	The lack of clarity or buy-in prevents team members from making decisions they will stick to
Fear of conflict	The desire to preserve artificial harmony stifles the occurrence of productive ideological conflict
Absence of trust	The fear of being vulnerable with team members prevents the building of trust within the team

We must remember that conflict is a normal part of professional work and should be accepted as something that WILL occur in the process of interacting with others. Conflict resolution training is common in health organisations and is considered essential for front-line workers in dealing with and de-escalating difficult and potentially dangerous situations with patients/carers. It is generally assumed that 'conflict' is negative, rather than seeing it as an opportunity for growth. However, the way we respond to and manage conflict is important to explore. Waite and McKinney (2014) suggest that nurses should develop purposeful conflict competence. This involves cognitive, emotional skills and behaviours to enhance productive outcomes of conflict, in addition to reducing the chance of harm/escalation. In order for teams to think differently about conflict, individuals must have a high level of self-awareness and understand their values in relation to others. There is a large evidence base relating to conflict competency in law and business, with healthcare disciplines drawing on these principles to develop communication strategies with leaders and teams. However, conflict competence goes further in relation to team dynamics. The fundamental message of slow down, reflect on the situation occurring, and collaborate constructively, reduces the risk of escalation.

You may not feel confident to deal with an underlying conflict where there are obvious personality clashes within the team. As you progress to a registered nurse and future leader of a team, you want to be fair to all parties, although other team members may voice their opinions to you. You will need to develop conflict competence over time, and you will not always get things right. However, the more exposure you have to conflict, the better you will become. Your team will also begin to understand and develop their own conflict competence if you promote collaborative learning. Constructive conflict can encourage creativity and innovation, stimulating change through discussions and resolving differences of opinions.

ACTIVITY 7.5

Think about your experiences of working within teams. How has conflict been managed? List behaviours and actions that were both positive and negative. What were the outcomes and how do you see each of the identified actions and behaviours contributing to these?

As suggested previously, conflict within teams needs to be approached constructively. It does not always present itself as purely verbal communication. It can be very subtle, often including non-verbal gestures such as tutting, eye rolling, yawning/showing signs of ignoring someone when they are speaking, closed body language, and dismissive comments to others. Demeaning, criticising and blaming behaviours are destructive in teams and can become personalised. Unhelpful strategies to manage conflict are avoiding the conflict or denying it exists, giving in to the person who shouts the loudest, and competing to win for your own benefit at all costs. A win–win collaborative solution is a positive strategy to encourage conflict competence. In order for this to be effective, the right climate and constructive communication needs to occur, as shown in *Table 7.4*.

Table 7.4 *Team conflict competence model (Runde and Flanagan, 2010)*

Right climate	**Constructive communication**
Attitudes	Reflective thinking and delayed responding
Trust	Listening for understanding
Safety	Perspective talking
Behavioural integration	Expressing emotions
Emotional intelligence	Techniques for staying on track

Given below is a four-step approach used within many NHS organisations. You may have seen or experienced this approach within your placement experiences.

1. Separate the person from the problem. It is important to focus on the problem that is causing the conflict. If someone's attitude or behaviour is causing the conflict, identify how this can be changed, not the person.
2. Focus on the underlying reasons for the demands, not necessarily on the demands themselves.
3. Consider creative solutions that meet the needs of both parties. Aim for what makes sense, rather than what is 'wanted'.
4. Identify objective criteria to ensure negotiations reach a fair conclusion and can be followed up with evaluation.

It is sometimes tempting to ignore the conflict around you because it is easier to pretend it isn't happening. However, always deal with conflict as soon as possible, if not immediately you become aware of the issue. Knowing you are open, trustworthy and will listen without pre-judging will help colleagues approach you as soon as they have an issue to raise. If not, the problem will be allowed to fester and become harder to resolve.

Practise clear, calm communication where your thoughts and ideas can be expressed without ambiguity and always check the receiver understands your message. You must also practise active listening as discussed in previous chapters, to clarify and question meaning, paraphrasing where appropriate.

Do not engage with elements of conflict that may involve personalities, although it is important to acknowledge attitude. Avoid blame and encourage ownership of the issue and possible solutions. Ask parties to use 'I' in explaining the issues rather than 'you'; for example, "I felt annoyed and upset because…." rather than "You always do things like this which….". This can only be accomplished if all parties are encouraged to be honest in expressing their views and feelings. Focus on the facts and issues raised, in particular what can be 'actioned' to change. Do not dwell on what cannot be changed.

Respect for all parties and their views must be a prerequisite for any conflict resolution discussion. Accept that you may need to call a break and reconvene if emotions escalate. Keep the meeting within the team and do not be tempted to discuss issues outside the parties involved unless further fact finding is necessary. Wider discussion can cause the conflict issues to build without being addressed directly.

7.7 Supervising others

Supervising others, such as junior student nurses, trainee nurse associates, HCAs and also new members of registered nursing staff once you are a registrant yourself, can be very rewarding and can benefit both development and professional socialisation. It helps to see this role as a *shared* learning journey where you can gain new knowledge, enhance skills, improve understanding and discuss situations and events with each other in order to improve patient care.

Johansson *et al.*'s (2010) study saw the supervisory relationship as the most important factor in determining the outcome of the clinical learning experience. This also corresponds to the views of mentors who feel they are the most important source of support in clinical practice (McIntosh *et al.*, 2013; Robinson, 2013). When supervising those who are with you for a limited time, this supervisory relationship requires building a trusting working relationship very quickly. As discussed in previous chapters, effective communication skills are essential within all learning and teaching situations to ensure a shared understanding of meaning that can be translated into actions. In order to promote conditions to facilitate a positive supervisory relationship, the following conditions must be considered:

- unconditional acceptance of the supervisee and mutual respect
- honesty and genuineness
- acknowledging and empathising with each other's viewpoints.

In addition to the above prerequisite conditions, the initial communication with the supervisee must be planned in advance. Time should be taken to find out their current experience and needs. For example, is this their first placement experience, do they have any learning needs or entitlements, are there any cultural needs that must be considered? You may want to contact the educational institute or practice facilitator/education lead for further information. It will help the supervisee feel valued that you have taken the time to retrieve some personal information.

Adequate time should be planned for the initial meeting to explain mandatory information such as safety processes and raising concerns. It is important to discuss expectations for you, the team and the supervisee, in addition to negotiating learning opportunities to facilitate necessary assessment requirements.

The supervisory relationship may require both authoritative and facilitative communication interventions, depending on the situations arising. *Table 7.5* shows Heron's (1989) six-category intervention analysis, which is relevant to consider here. Although the model was originally developed for counselling mediation, it is often used when planning and reflecting on communication episodes with individuals and teams. In the supervisory relationship, the supervisor can choose which category is most appropriate for the situation.

Table 7.5 *Six-category intervention analysis (Heron, 1989)*

Authoritative intervention	Facilitative intervention
Prescriptive: giving advice and direction	Cathartic: encouraging and allowing expression of emotions
Informative: giving information to guide and direct	Catalytic: encouraging reflection and deeper learning to become more self-directed
Confrontational: directly challenge, positively and constructively (not aggressively)	Supportive: building confidence, encouraging and understanding

ACTIVITY 7.6

Consider the six-category intervention analysis in *Table 7.5*. Think of possible situations you may come across in a supervisory arrangement where you could use each of the interventions. You may want to draw on your own experience as a supervisee.

Which do you feel are the most comfortable to use and why?

Which ones do you feel may prove more challenging to use and why?

Devise a checklist of the requirements you feel would be necessary to ensure a positive supervisory relationship.

Many nurses in supervisory roles find it easier to teach a skill or task, but find it difficult to 'teach' professional values. Consequently, this needs to be communicated in alternative ways such as role modelling, reflective discussion, case study examples, and considering how the NMC *Code* is translated to practice scenarios. You may also want to direct students and supervisees to reviewed electronic sources to provide visual and audio clips relating to professional identity. In order to build confidence in supervisees and embed professional considerations, you could consider a coaching model. Coaching is concerned with helping an individual or group learn and unlock their potential for growth and development, rather than 'teaching' them (Narayanasamy and Penny, 2014). The GROW coaching model (see *Figure 7.3*) can be used to structure practice learning and incorporate professional socialisation.

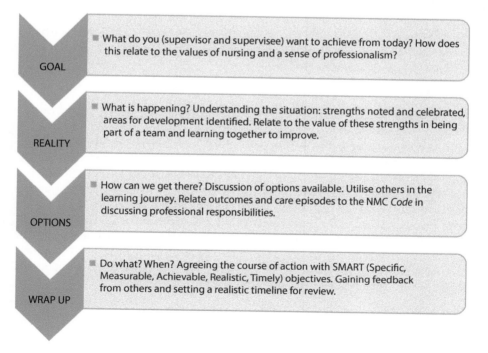

GOAL — What do you (supervisor and supervisee) want to achieve from today? How does this relate to the values of nursing and a sense of professionalism?

REALITY — What is happening? Understanding the situation: strengths noted and celebrated, areas for development identified. Relate to the value of these strengths in being part of a team and learning together to improve.

OPTIONS — How can we get there? Discussion of options available. Utilise others in the learning journey. Relate outcomes and care episodes to the NMC *Code* in discussing professional responsibilities.

WRAP UP — Do what? When? Agreeing the course of action with SMART (Specific, Measurable, Achievable, Realistic, Timely) objectives. Gaining feedback from others and setting a realistic timeline for review.

Figure 7.3 *Adapted from the GROW coaching model (Passmore, 2006).*

In any supervisory relationship, giving constructive, honest feedback that promotes development and improvement is essential. This is how your supervisee will progress and learn. However, it can be difficult giving feedback when areas for improvement have been identified. Nevertheless, as a supervisor or coach you must remember to give feedback that is specific to help the supervisee understand and clarify the particular areas that require focus to improve. It is common to use general terms such as: "That wasn't too bad…", "That's OK but could be a bit better….", "That's not quite to standard as yet….", "Keep practising….", yet this can be confusing for the supervisee and does not clearly identify the areas requiring further development.

In the model below, Jerome (1999) describes four stages of feedback relating to coaching. This can be used to plan and structure the feedback for your supervisee. Remember to ask others who have been involved in working with your supervisee to ensure the feedback includes views and comments from a range of relevant sources.

1. Provide a description of current behaviours that you want to reinforce and redirect to improve a situation.
2. Identify specific situations where these behaviours have been observed.
3. Describe impacts and consequences of the current behaviours.
4. Identify alternative behaviours and actions that can be taken.

CASE STUDY

You are a newly qualified staff nurse starting your first post as a registrant. Your peers have talked about this placement in a very negative way, suggesting you will not feel part of a team and that the communication between staff is poor. You try not to pre-judge and decide to make the most of the learning opportunities available. As a registrant you hope to continue linking theory you have gained from your studies, relating to communication and teamwork, to encourage a change in practice.

Following your first week, you reflect on the issues that have occurred.

Your preceptor, Jay, was off sick for the first four days of your placement. The team were therefore short-staffed and you tried to help as much as possible by speaking initially with the ward manager to identify your current level of competence and the skills you felt could be utilised. The ward manager was very grateful and apologised for not being able to allocate another preceptor. She asked you to work alongside a specific HCA for a few days to get used to the ward environment. However, the named HCA had previously been asked to work with a registered nurse to care for a patient with particularly complex needs. She said you would need to speak with the ward manager again, who was nowhere to be found on ward and no one knew why. Multiple conversations were happening with various team members but there was no overall team meeting or overall team communication. You felt frustrated at the lack of teamwork and communication and could see how patient care was being affected.

What action points would you consider following this first week?

Your preceptor Jay returned and your next few weeks saw similar communication issues. Jay and the ward manager did not communicate with each other unless absolutely necessary. It became apparent that they had completed their nurse education together, although Jay felt she had not achieved the relevant promotions because she 'stood up for her patients' and was therefore seen as a trouble-maker. Jay told you the ward manager was promoted beyond her competence and she had no respect for her. This continued and you felt uncomfortable hearing information about a colleague in this way. No team meetings were held in this first month. Allocation of patient care was not organised efficiently, with some staff being allocated to patients with very complex needs, while others had only a few patients who were mainly self-caring.

What action points would you consider to address these issues?

During your second month you were allocated to work with a first-year student nurse for the week who appeared very worried at being allocated this placement. You discussed how theory could link to this practice area and asked the student to identify her goals for this learning opportunity. You enjoyed working with the student and, together with her overarching assessor, discussed how feedback should be organised. Her nominated supervisor was happy to write some comments in her assessment document as she did not have the time to arrange a face-to-face meeting with the student.

What action points would you consider following this decision?

What would be your short-term and long-term action points going forward?

Summary

Effective communication in teamworking can be influenced by many factors, including interpersonal relationships, leadership, organisational culture, agreed goals and sharing information. The underpinning focus must always be the quality care of patients and/or communities. It may not be an easy process to achieve, as discussed above; however, there are many strategies, tools and models that can be used to assist in working through potential difficulties. It is our professional responsibility to challenge poor practice, encourage the resolving of differences, respect our colleagues, and work together to achieve high standards of care and service delivery.

KEY LEARNING POINTS

Four key points to take away from *Chapter 7*:
- ☑ An open, transparent, strengths-based approach to teamwork is needed for effective care delivery.
- ☑ Take time to know your immediate team and colleagues from the wider healthcare provision, including their specific roles, in order to plan and influence negotiation strategies.
- ☑ As a future leader of nursing care delivery, be aware of strategies to create positive cultures in the workplace. Listen to staff and role model behaviours to encourage trust, respect and care excellence.
- ☑ Adopt a coaching approach to supervisory relationships with nursing students. This builds confidence, encourages specific solution-focused action points, and develops shared learning.

FURTHER READING

Clouston, T.J., Westcott, L. and Whitcombe, S.W. (2018) *Transitions to Practice: essential concepts for health and social care professions*. M&K Publishing.

Gopee, N. and Galloway, J. (2017) *Leadership and Management in Healthcare*, 3rd edition. Sage.

Jones, L. and Bennett, C. (2018) *Leadership: for nursing, health and social care students*. Lantern Publishing Ltd.

Raphael-Grimm, T. (2014) *The Art of Communication in Nursing and Health Care: an interdisciplinary approach*. Springer Publishing Company.

Schein, E.H. (2016) *Organisational Culture and Leadership*, 5th edition. John Wiley & Sons, Inc.

Sennett, R. (2012) *Together: the rituals, pleasures and politics of cooperation*. Yale University Press.

REFERENCES

Belbin, R.M. (2010) *Team Roles at Work*. Routledge.

Bhatt, A. and Mitchell, A. (2015) Effective collaborative communication in hospice care. *Palliative Medicine and Care*, **2(1)**: 1–13.

Cornell, P. and Townsend-Gervis, M. (2014) Improving situation awareness and patient outcomes through interdisciplinary rounding and structured communication. *The Journal of Nursing Administration*, **44(3)**: 164–9.

Curtis, E.A. and Cullen, J.G. (eds) (2017) *Leadership and Change for the Health Professional*. Open University Press.

Dixon-Woods, M., Baker, R., Charles, K. *et al.* (2014) Culture and behaviour in the English National Health Service: overview of lessons from a large multimethod study. *BMJ Quality and Safety*, **23(2)**: 106–15.

Forsyth, P. (2009) *Negotiation Skills for Rookies*. Marshall Cavendish.

Francis, R. (chair) (2013) *Report of the Mid Staffordshire NHS Foundation Trust Public Inquiry*. The Stationery Office. Available at: https://assets.publishing. service.gov.uk/government/uploads/system/uploads/attachment_data/ file/279124/0947.pdf (accessed 19 July 2019).

Hammond, W. (2010) *Principles of Strength-Based Practice*. Resiliency Initiatives. Available at: https://greaterfallsconnections.org/wp-content/uploads/2014/07/Principles-of-Strength-2.pdf (accessed 19 July 2019).

Heron, J. (1989) *Six-Category Intervention Analysis*, 3rd edition. Human Potential Research Group, University of Surrey.

Hunter, B. and Warren, L. (2013) *Investigating Resilience in Midwifery*. Final Report. Cardiff University. Available at: https://orca.cf.ac.uk/61594/1/Investigating%20resilience%20Final%20report%20oct%202013.pdf (accessed 19 July 2019).

Jerome, P.J. (1999) *Coaching Through Effective Feedback*. Pfeiffer Publishing.

Johansson, U-B., Kaila, P., Ahlner-Elmqvist, M. *et al*. (2010) Clinical learning environment, supervision and nurse teacher evaluation scale: psychometric evaluation of the Swedish version. *Journal of Advanced Nursing*, **66(9)**: 2085–93.

Karam, L., Brault, I., Van Durme, T. and Macq, J. (2018) Comparing interprofessional and interorganizational collaboration in healthcare: a systematic review of the qualitative research. *International Journal of Nursing Studies*, **79**: 70–83.

King's Fund (2016) *Crossing Professional Boundaries: a toolkit for collaborative working*. Available at: www.futurefocusedfinance.nhs.uk/crossing-professional-boundaries-toolkit (accessed 19 July 2019).

Lancaster, G., Kolakowsky-Hayner, S., Kovacich, J. and Greer-Williams, N. (2015) Interdisciplinary communication and collaboration among physicians, nurses, and unlicensed assistive personnel. *Nursing Scholarship*, **47(3)**: 275–84.

Lencioni, P. (2009) *The Five Dysfunctions of a Team*. Jossey-Bass.

McIntosh, A., Gidman, J. and Smith, D. (2013) Mentors' perceptions and experiences of supporting student nurses in practice. *International Journal of Nursing Practice*, **20**: 360–5.

Miles, E. and Trott, W. (2011) *Collaborative Working*. Institute for Government. Available at: www.instituteforgovernment.org.uk/sites/default/files/publications/Collaborative%20working.pdf (accessed 19 July 2019).

Narayanasamy, A. and Penny, V. (2014) Coaching to promote professional development in nursing practice. *British Journal of Nursing*, **23(11)**: 568–73.

NHS England (2014) *Building and Strengthening Leadership: leading with compassion*. NHS England. Available at: www.england.nhs.uk/wp-content/uploads/2014/12/london-nursing-accessible.pdf (accessed 19 July 2019).

NHS Leadership Academy (2017) *Developing Better Leaders, Delivering Better Care*. Available at: www.leadershipacademy.nhs.uk (accessed 19 July 2019).

Nursing and Midwifery Council (2018) *The Code: professional standards of practice and behaviour for nurses, midwives and nursing associates*. NMC. Available at: www.nmc.org.uk/globalassets/sitedocuments/nmc-publications/nmc-code.pdf (accessed 19 July 2019).

Passmore, J. (2006) *Excellence in Coaching: the industry guide*. Kogan Page.

Radtke, K. (2013) Improving patient satisfaction with nursing communication using bedside shift report. *Clinical Nurse Specialist*, **27(1)**: 19–25.

Robinson, S. (2013) Sustaining mentorship for student nurses. *Nursing Times*, **109**: 24–5.

Runde, C.E. and Flanagan, T.A. (2010) *Developing your Conflict Competence: a hands-on guide for leaders, managers, facilitators, and teams*. Jossey-Bass/The Center for Creative Leadership.

Waite, R. and McKinney, M.S. (2014) Enhancing conflict competency. *ABNF Journal*, **25(4)**: 123–8.

West, M., Dawson, J., Admasachew, L. and Topakas, A. (2011) *NHS Staff Management and Health Service Quality: results from the NHS staff survey and related data*. Department of Health. Available at: https://assets.publishing.service.gov.uk/government/uploads/system/uploads/attachment_data/file/215455/dh_129656.pdf (accessed 19 July 2019).

Chapter 8
Communication for patient safety

Val Nixon

LEARNING OUTCOMES

By the end of this chapter you should be able to:

8.1 Understand the concepts of patient safety and how the implementation of patient safety initiatives has influenced current patient safety practices

8.2 Appreciate the multifaceted dimensions of safety culture and the role of effective communication in promoting a positive safety culture

8.3 Apply the principles of human factors to recognise how patient safety incidents occur in healthcare practice

8.4 Reflect upon the importance of incident reporting and strategies you and other healthcare professionals can use to learn from incidents.

8.1 Introduction

Effective communication is key to patient safety to ensure no harm occurs in the delivery of patient care. Nurses constitute the largest workforce in the NHS and play a vital role in ensuring patient safety, spending the most time with patients and performing many roles. These include providing effective and safe care, ongoing patient monitoring and coordination of care. Protecting patients from harm can be seen as fundamental in all nursing activities.

Generally, the vast majority of patients accessing healthcare services will have a positive experience due to the high-quality, safe care delivered by dedicated healthcare professionals. However, errors and omissions in their care result in harm to some patients and most of these incidents are preventable. In a review of root cause analyses, communication was found to be an important causal factor (World Health Organization, 2008) and is one of the most common causes of dissatisfaction within healthcare services (Royal College of Nursing, 2017).

Communication strategies are indicated in varying forms, as policies and procedures, performance statistics, incident reports, workplace inductions, learning from errors, education and training. These strategies are essential to engage healthcare professionals in patient safety activities that promote a positive safety culture. This chapter will provide an overview of patient safety and safety culture, and how human factor principles are applied to patient safety. The importance of learning from errors cannot be underestimated as this is key to promoting a positive safety culture. This relies, however, on effective incident reporting structures and strategies to support this process. Throughout this chapter, the term error will be applied to a patient safety incident where appropriate.

8.2 **Development of patient safety**

Patient safety has received global attention since the publication of *To Err is Human: building a safer health system* (Kohn *et al.*, 2000). The report estimated that 44 000–98 000 patients in the USA die each year as a direct result of medical errors that could have been prevented. In 2000, the UK equivalent *An Organisation with a Memory* (Department of Health, 2000) was published. This reported a poor record for patient safety in the NHS and estimated that every year (Department of Health, 2000, pp. vii–viii):

- 400 people die or are seriously injured in adverse events involving medical devices.
- Nearly 10 000 people are reported to have experienced serious adverse reactions to drugs.
- Around 1150 people who have been in recent contact with mental health services take their own life.
- Nearly 28 000 written complaints are made about aspects of clinical treatment in hospitals.
- The NHS pays out around £400 million a year for the settlement of clinical negligence claims and has a potential liability of around £2.4 billion for existing and expected claims.
- Hospital-acquired infections – around 15% of which may be avoidable – are estimated to cost the NHS nearly £1 billion.
- Adverse events in NHS hospitals, where harm is caused to patients, occur in around 10% of admissions – or at a rate in excess of 850 000 a year.
- The cost to the NHS as a result of harm is estimated at £2 billion a year in additional hospital stays alone. This cost does not take into account any additional human or wider economic costs (e.g. for loss of earnings to those who are harmed, clinical negligence claims).

This landmark report paved the way for a national programme of action across the UK to improve patient safety, which is illustrated in *Table 8.1*. Despite implementation of these national developments, patient safety continues to be a national priority as the number of patient safety incidents continues to increase. The number of incidents reported from October to December 2017 (via the National Reporting and Learning System, NRLS) were 508 409. This is a five-fold increase since 2005, when the numbers reported were 135 356 (NHS Improvement, 2018).

Table 8.1 *Chronology of national developments related to patient safety in England 2000–2018 (adapted from The Health Foundation, 2013)*

Year	National developments
2001	Establishment of the National Patient Safety Agency (NPSA)
2001	Mandatory reporting of methicillin-resistant *Staphylococcus aureus* (MRSA)
2003	National Reporting and Learning System (NRLS) implemented to capture all adverse events reported in the NHS in England and Wales
2004	Safer Patients Initiative (collaborative partnership with the Institute for Healthcare Improvement [IHI] in the USA)
2004	Healthcare Commission – to assess standards of care provided by the NHS
2005	Saving Lives – to reduce harm caused by MRSA and *Clostridium difficile*
2009	Care Quality Commission (CQC) took over from the Healthcare Commission. The CQC regulates all health and social care services in England (see www.cqc.org.uk)
2009	Introduction of Commissioning for Quality and Innovation (CQUIN) national goals, to secure improvements in the quality of services and better outcomes against national goals (www.england.nhs.uk/wp-content/uploads/2016/03/cquin-guidance-16-17-v3.pdf)
2010	NHS Outcomes Framework published by the Department of Health with two of the five domains central to patient safety
2012	Quality, Innovation, Productivity and Prevention (QIPP) developed the NHS Safety Thermometer CQUIN (NHS ST) to incentivise the measurement of harm from falls, urinary infection in patients with indwelling catheters, pressure ulcers and venous thromboembolism risk assessment (see www.safetythermometer.nhs.uk)
2016	NHS Improvement responsible for overseeing NHS Foundation Trusts, NHS Trusts and independent providers, helping them to give patients consistently safe, high-quality care within local health systems (see https://improvement.nhs.uk)
2015	The Nursing and Midwifery Council (NMC) introduced patient safety into *The Code: professional standards of practice and behaviour for nurses and midwives* (revised in 2018 to reflect introduction of nursing associates)
2018	The NMC (2018b) introduced patient safety into their new *Future Nurse: standards of proficiency for registered nurses*. This reflects the contribution that nurses make to continuously monitor and improve quality of care that will enhance health outcomes

8.2.1 Concept of patient safety

At its simplest, patient safety is defined as the "prevention of patient harm" (Kohn *et al.*, 2000). The World Health Organization (2009, p. 15) offers a similar but broader definition and states that: "Patient safety is the reduction of risk of unnecessary harm associated with healthcare to an acceptable minimum."

The use of the word 'unnecessary' in this definition recognises that errors, violation, patient abuse and deliberate unsafe acts (termed 'incidents') occur in healthcare. To standardise the terms used relating to incidents, the World Health Organization (2009) has published an International Classification for Patient Safety (ICPS). This conceptual framework was developed to enable categorisation of patient safety information by using a standardised set of concepts and agreed definitions. *Table 8.2* illustrates some examples of the key concepts and definitions commonly used in clinical practice.

Table 8.2 *Key concepts and definitions (World Health Organization, 2009)*

Concept	Definition
Event	Something that happened to or involved a patient
Healthcare-associated harm	Harm arising from or associated with plans or actions taken during the provision of healthcare, rather than an underlying disease or injury
Patient safety incident	An event or circumstance that could have resulted, or did result, in unnecessary harm to a patient; these arise from violation or error
Violation	**Intended acts** due to deliberate deviation from a procedure or standard or rule
Error	**Unintentional acts** due to failure to carry out planned action as intended or application of an incorrect plan. Errors may manifest by doing the wrong thing (commission) or by failing to do the right thing (omission), at either the planning or execution phase
Harm	Implies impairment of structure or function of the body and/or damaging effect arising therefrom, including disease, injury, suffering, disability and death, and may be physical, social or psychological

While healthcare brings enormous benefits to those using the health service, errors are common, and patients are frequently harmed. It is important to recognise that healthcare and healthcare delivery is a multifaceted phenomenon reflected by the complexities of health, social, political and organisational context (Curry and Nunez-Smith, 2015). Individual beliefs, values and motivations that underlie individual behaviours are also complex, and therefore keeping patients safe from harm is a significant issue and one of the most prominent healthcare challenges worldwide. As previously outlined (see *Table 8.1*), there has been an increasing focus in the UK (and internationally) on improving patient safety and this has led to greater recognition of the importance of the safety culture of organisations and teams, particularly with regard to how communication can be improved.

8.2.2 Safety culture

'Safety culture' is integral to the overall culture of an organisation. The following definition of safety culture was originally cited in the UK Health and Safety

Commission report in 1993 and is quoted widely in the healthcare literature and many government reports:

> The safety culture of an organisation is the product of the individual and group values, attitudes, competencies and patterns of behaviour that determine the commitment to, and the style and proficiency of, an organisation's health and safety programmes…

(cited in Health Foundation, 2013, p. 5)

Safety culture as a concept is usually described in terms of perceptions relating to trust, values and attitudes that focus upon preventing errors and maintaining patient safety. It also refers to the way in which patient safety is thought about, how this is implemented within an organisation, and the structures and processes in place to support this. All these factors have a huge positive or negative influence on patient safety outcomes. The effect of a healthcare organisation's safety culture on patient clinical outcomes has been studied extensively, with communication identified as an important organisational aspect affecting patient safety (Wang *et al.*, 2014). A positive safety culture is therefore characterised by effective communication founded on mutual trust to keep patients safe from actual and potential harm. In comparison, a negative safety culture can cause harm and injury and can be characterised by poor communication of patient safety issues within clinical environments and across the organisations. *Table 8.3* provides further characteristics that you may experience in your clinical practice areas.

Table 8.3 *Examples of positive and negative characteristics associated with safety culture*

Positive safety culture	Negative safety culture
<ul><li>Good communication up, down and across the organisation</li><li>A positive attitude towards risk management</li><li>Good reporting systems</li><li>Willingness to report errors</li><li>Willingness to learn from errors to bring about continual improvement</li><li>Blame-free culture</li><li>Visible management and commitment at all levels</li><li>Shared perceptions of the importance of safety</li><li>Workforce involvement in all aspects of patient safety so each individual feels responsible for the safety of their patients</li></ul>	<ul><li>Lack of communication</li><li>Risk assessments: risk and consequences not seen as a priority when they actually are</li><li>Poor or inadequate reporting system</li><li>Infrequency of reporting errors</li><li>Inadequate analyses of adverse events</li><li>Lack of feedback and communication about errors</li><li>Blame culture at all levels of the organisation</li><li>Poor leadership and management decisions</li><li>Education and training given low priority and over-reliance on e-training</li></ul>

In general, the overall concept of safety culture focuses upon preventing errors and maintaining patient safety, which may seem straightforward. However, promoting a positive safety culture is multifaceted due to the different dimensions that are associated with it. The Agency for Healthcare Research and Quality (AHRQ) identified

12 dimensions (as described and defined in *Table 8.4*) when it developed the Hospital Survey on Patient Safety Culture (HSOPSC). This is a pre-validated questionnaire that is widely used internationally to study and evaluate individual perceptions of safety culture in hospital settings (AHRQ, 2012). Other pre-validated questionnaires such as the Safety Attitude Questionnaire (SAQ) (developed by Sexton *et al.*, 2006) also identify similar dimensions. It is beyond the remit of this chapter to discuss safety culture questionnaires in detail. Further information can be found on The Health Foundation website (www.health.org.uk/sites/default/files/MeasuringSafetyCulture.pdf). This document provides a summary of the surveys, together with their strengths and weaknesses.

ACTIVITY 8.1

Take time to review the safety culture dimensions and descriptions in *Table 8.4*. Can you see how they predominantly relate to communication?

Now go to page 40 of the Hospital Survey on Patient Safety Culture (HOSPSC), which can be accessed here: bit.ly/HOSPSC-40 or by scanning the QR code on the right.

Consider your experience of safety culture within two different clinical areas, then complete the survey for each placement and compare your responses.

Consider any individual, team and organisational factors that have influenced your perceptions relating to your responses.

Table 8.4 *Dimensions and definition of safety culture dimensions (AHRQ, 2012)*

Patient safety culture dimension	Definition: The extent to which...
Communication	Staff freely speak up if they see something that may negatively affect a patient and feel free to question those with more authority
Feedback and communication about error	Staff are informed about errors that happen, are given feedback about changes implemented, and discuss ways to prevent errors
Frequency of event reported	Mistakes of the following types are reported 1. Mistakes caught and corrected before affecting the patient 2. Mistakes with no potential harm 3. Mistakes that could harm the patient but do not
Patient handover and transitions	Important patient care information is transferred on admission/discharge and during shift changes

(continued)

Table 8.4 *(continued)*

Patient safety culture dimension	Definition: The extent to which…
Management support for patient safety	Hospital management provides a work climate that promotes patient safety and shows that patient safety is a top priority
Non-punitive response to error	Staff feel that their mistakes and event reports are not held against them and mistakes are not kept in their personal file
Organisational learning – continuous improvement	Mistakes have led to positive changes and changes are evaluated for effectiveness
Overall perceptions of patient safety	Procedures and systems are good at preventing errors and there is a lack of patient safety problems
Staffing	There are enough staff to handle the workload and work hours are appropriate to provide the best care for patients
Supervisor/manager expectations and actions promoting patient safety	Supervisors/managers consider staff suggestions for improving patient safety problems
Teamwork across the organisation	Organisations cooperate with one another to provide the best care for patients
Teamwork within individual clinical environments	Staff support each other, treat each other with respect, and work together as a team

8.3 Incident reporting

Since the publication of *An Organisation with a Memory* (Department of Health, 2000), healthcare organisations have made significant efforts to reduce patient safety incidents and subsequent harm. It is now recognised that an organisation's safety culture and approach to patient safety incidents are key factors influencing safety and quality. As a form of communication, incident reporting is an established mechanism for improving patient safety. Organisations with a positive safety culture (as illustrated in *Table 8.3*) report a large number of patient safety incidents and acknowledge healthcare professionals for their candour and commitment to learning. In comparison, those organisations with a negative safety culture will blame individuals and consider reporting those incidents 'out of line' (Taylor, 2012). It is important to note that an increased number of reported patient safety incidents reflects an improved reporting culture and should not be interpreted as a decrease in the safety of the NHS. Equally, a decrease cannot be interpreted as an increase in the safety of the NHS.

Evidence suggests that there is a positive correlation between safety incident reporting data and a high Hospital Mortality Ratio Score (HMRS) for those organisations that report large numbers of incidents (Keogh, 2013). Conversely, it is recognised that only a relatively small percentage of incidents that occur are actually reported. In addition, those incidents that are considered 'near misses' were not reported. In nursing, the reasons for failure to report incidents have been extensively researched (for example, Alahmadi, 2010; El-Jardali *et al.*, 2014) and findings reveal a number of barriers to reporting, for example:

- time constraints
- failure to recognise an incident
- feeling threatened
- fear of blame
- failure to receive feedback.

Any patient safety incident is a reportable circumstance where there is significant potential for harm, near miss or no harm (adverse event) for one or more patients receiving healthcare. Another key challenge when reporting a patient safety incident is the terminology that is used within the reporting systems. *Table 8.5* (in conjunction with *Table 8.2*) provides further descriptions of terminology used, together with an example for each classification of incident. As a student or registered nurse, you will encounter unintended or unexpected patient safety incidents in your placement experiences and it is fundamental that you "demonstrate an understanding of how to identify, report and critically reflect on near misses, critical incidents, major incidents and serious adverse events in order to learn from them and influence their future practice" (NMC, 2018b, p. 22).

Figure 8.1 demonstrates the process that should be followed when patient safety incidents occur.

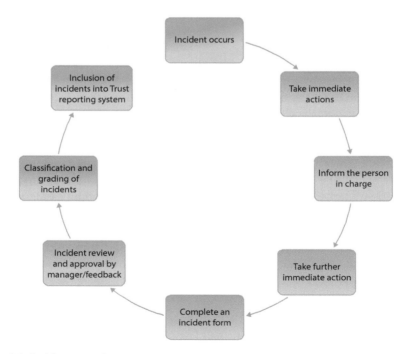

Figure 8.1 *Incident reporting process.*

8.3.1 Incident reporting systems

ALL patient safety incidents must be recorded on the local risk management system. The Datix is an electronic incident reporting and risk management system that is widely used in health and social care organisations across the UK. Staff training has become part of the mandatory and statutory training for NHS Trusts. Datix reports feed into the National Reporting and Learning System (NRLS). The NRLS is the world's largest and most comprehensive patient safety incident reporting system and receives over two million reports each year. It is managed and operated by NHS Improvement as part of its statutory duty to collect patient safety incident reports. Healthcare organisations, staff and the general public can also record patient safety incidents directly to the NRLS using electronic forms available on the NRLS website (https://improvement.nhs.uk/resources/report-patient-safety-incident/).

NHS Improvement has developed a two-minute video outlining the importance of reporting patient safety incidents to the NRLS, which you can access at https://improvement.nhs.uk/resources/learning-from-patient-safety-incidents/

Table 8.5 *Classification of incidents (adapted from World Health Organization, 2009)*

Classification	Description	Example
A harmful incident (also referred to as an adverse incident)	A patient safety incident that resulted in harm to a patient, including harm resulting when a patient did not receive their planned or expected treatment	Managing a deteriorating patient. Failure to record and monitor Early Warning Scores and the patient died of sepsis
A no harm incident	A patient safety incident occurred but did not result in patient harm	Patient falling in the corridor and no reported injuries following examination
A near miss	A patient safety incident that did not reach the patient but had the potential to do so	Antibiotics prescribed to a patient. On administrating the drug to the patient, they inform you of their allergy to antibiotics. The error is detected before this drug is administered

When reporting, the patient incident type and grading of that patient safety incident should be recorded. The patient incident type is a descriptive term for a category of a common nature; for example, failing to monitor a patient will be categorised as implementation of care and ongoing monitoring/review; 'medication/IV fluid' would be categorised as medication. Although each incident type concept is distinct, a patient safety incident can be classified as more than one incident type. The grading of patient safety incidents relates to the patient outcome, i.e. the impact upon a patient that is wholly or partially attributable to the patient safety incident. Patient outcomes can be classified according to the degree of harm and any social and/or economic impact. The degree of harm is the severity and duration of any harm and any treatment implications, which are described in *Table 8.6*. In order to prioritise clinical reviews, recording the degree of harm is not only crucial for prioritising clinical reviews of these patient safety incidents, but critical to encourage learning. This enables healthcare professionals to identify those patient safety incidents causing most harm, and more importantly, to learn about the impact this has on patients and their families (see *Activity 8.4*).

Table 8.6 *Categories of degree of harm (NHS Improvement, 2018, p. 12)*

Degree of harm	Description
No harm	A situation where no harm occurred: either a prevented patient safety incident or a no harm incident
Low harm	Any unexpected incident that required extra observation or minor treatment and caused minimal harm to one or more persons
Moderate harm	Any unexpected or unintended incident that resulted in further treatment, possible surgical intervention, cancelling of treatment, or transfer to another area, and which caused short-term harm to one or more persons
Severe harm	Any unexpected or unintended incident that caused permanent or long-term harm to one or more persons
Death	Any unexpected or unintended event that caused the death of one or more persons

8.4 A human factors approach to patient safety

The NMC (2018a, p. 17) states that you must "take account of current evidence, knowledge and developments in reducing mistakes and the effect of them and the impact on human factors and system failures".

In healthcare, the principles of human factors are now widely used as a key element in improving patient safety (Berwick, 2013). The human factors approach to patient safety is derived from the aviation industry and is widely used in many other safety-critical industries such as rail transport, petrochemical plants and nuclear power plants. Safety-critical industries are those industries in which safety is of paramount importance and where the consequences of failure or malfunction may be loss of life or serious injury, serious environmental damage, or harm to plant or property (Wears, 2012). The lessons and examples from these industries (as a result of major accidents) have shown that using human factors principles in healthcare delivery can improve work processes. It helps to understand how healthcare systems can minimise unavoidable errors and patient harm, for example by applying safe prescribing practices, promoting effective communication within teams, and handing over information to other healthcare professionals.

Human factors (often referred to as ergonomics) can be defined in many ways but a widely accepted definition is that of the Health and Safety Executive (1999, p. 5): "Human factors refer to environmental, organisational and job factors, and human and individual characteristics which influence behaviour at work in a way which can affect health and safety."

Human factors is an established scientific discipline that applies elements of other disciplines such as psychology, anatomy and physiology, social sciences, engineering, design and organisational management. It combines these disciplines to better understand the nature of human–technology–systems interactions. A system refers to something that can be designed to make it easy to do the right thing, or conversely, make it difficult to get things wrong. Examples of the types of systems in healthcare include:

- clinical tools (for example, a range of patient assessment tools)
- medication safety processes (e.g. for medicine administration)
- local and national clinical protocols and guidelines
- effective communication
- medical devices
- patient monitoring equipment
- education and training
- patient engagement (e.g. Patient Advice and Liaison Service (PALS), patient satisfaction surveys).

A major source of risk in healthcare lies within the system surrounding and interacting with those who deliver direct patient care. The human factors approach to patient safety starts with an understanding of the relationship of those systems that may support or hinder the way people work. It also explores the interplay between the healthcare staff providing care (people and culture) and the organisational and clinical contexts in which this care is delivered (systems and processes). *Figure 8.2* demonstrates the interaction of human factors and examples of key characteristics that make up the workplace system.

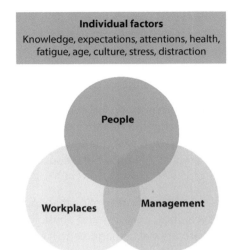

Figure 8.2 *Interaction of human factors and key characteristics for each dimension.*

8.4.1 A human factors approach to patient safety incidents

Delivering nursing care is dynamic and often carried out in unpredictable circumstances, for a variety of reasons. This may include the number of patients and their clinical condition, working conditions, staff workload and staff shortages, etc. This can put pressure on nurses, teams and organisations, which can directly impact on the quality of care, clinical outcomes and potentially lead to a patient safety incident.

Nursing care delivery is dependent on human beings and people think that safety lies foremost in the hands through which nursing care is delivered; the 'sharp end'. This is not surprising, considering that the clinical setting is fundamentally where patient safety occurs, where nurse–patient interaction occurs, where failures of safety emerge, and where patients are harmed (Brasaite *et al.*, 2015). Yet, the whole healthcare team can be involved in a patient safety incident, but the nurse is often at the 'sharp end' of the problem, the last step prior to reaching the patient. It is tempting to see human error as the cause and subsequently easy to blame that individual. Nevertheless, when patient safety incidents in nursing care occur, there is a human factors element present. The basic principle is that nurses are human, and humans are fallible, and so well-intentioned people do make unintended mistakes and/or are involved in systems that have failed around them. Human error, nonetheless, is a starting point, and it is important to explore all the causal factors that may have contributed to the patient safety incident. Supporting, not blaming, individuals is critical, so mistakes and the system failings will be reported to encourage learning from them (Berwick, 2013).

ACTIVITY 8.2

You are administering medications under the supervision of a registered nurse (RN). You have administered a prescribed dose of digoxin to Mrs Smith, when the RN is called away to answer the telephone. The RN locks the medication trolley and proceeds to answer the telephone before you sign the prescription chart. You did not sign the prescription chart as the RN needs to countersign your signature. The RN returns to find you assisting a patient to the toilet, so she proceeds to complete the medication round. When you return, you notice that she has administered another dose of digoxin.

Consider the individual, the workplace and the organisation in this scenario. Using a human errors approach, list the contributory factors relating to this patient safety incident.

8.5 **Learning from errors**

An important responsibility and requirement for any organisation is the ability to learn from errors. Identifying common factors that contribute to errors is critical to the development of solutions to promote a safer environment. Many factors contribute to errors and human errors occur for a variety of known and complicated reasons. When things go wrong, we often see that multiple things within the system led to the point that someone at the 'sharp end' got it wrong. When this happens, we have to distinguish between active failures and latent failures (Reason, 1997) as described below.

8.5.1 **Active failure (or active error)**

This describes unsafe acts or conditions precipitating the incident and usually committed by those at the 'sharp end' of the system. The consequences are immediate and can often be prevented.

8.5.2 **Latent failure (or latent errors)**

This describes less apparent failures of organisation or design that contribute to the occurrence of errors. They may lie dormant for days, weeks or months, only becoming evident when they combine with local triggering factors within the workplace (for example time, understaffing, fatigue and inexperience).

Example: The nurse administered the wrong drug to a patient. In this instance, the ward is busy; the nurse undertaking the medication round is at the end of a 12-hour shift and tired; the nurse is distracted because a patient is trying to climb out of bed; when administering the patient's drug, the nurse does not notice the similar packaging of two drugs that are stored close to each other.

As you can see from this example, the human factors principles can be applied to analyse the incident to identify what went wrong so that learning and corrective actions can take place. If we look at the above examples using 'the tip of the iceberg' model – what you see (the tip of the iceberg) is the nurse making the error (active failure). The larger part of the iceberg is below the surface and cannot be seen (latent failure). In this example, the active failure (nurse administering the wrong medication) is normally considered a small part of a bigger problem, because the latent failures include a busy ward, fatigue, distraction, different medication but similar packaging. These are factors that are contributory to this patient safety incident and are termed the root causes. If you compare this to the previous example in *Activity 8.2*, how does this differ? Are the root causes different? Or are they similar?

The root cause(s) are the most fundamental reason (or one of several reasons) for errors. To establish the root cause of a patient safety incident, a root cause analysis (RCA) must be undertaken. An RCA is the "systematic analysis of all the factors which predisposed to or had the potential to prevent an error" (World Health Organization, 2008, p. 18), and is the most widely deployed error analysis tool in healthcare. It focuses on a positive, preventative approach through applying the human factors principles to explain how the incident occurred. Systems and processes can then be redesigned to prevent it from happening again.

The simplest way to perform an RCA is to ask **why** five times, so you can peel away the layers of the problem to get to the root cause. This can be done by yourself, in teams, or it can be used to complement a thorough RCA.

ACTIVITY 8.3

In the example above, the questions might read as follows:
- Why was the nurse administering medication at the end of a 12-hour shift?
- Why was the patient climbing out of bed?
- Why was the ward busy?
- Why wasn't another member of staff there to assist the patient?
- Why wasn't the medication packaging clearly labelled for easy identification?

Consider the following questions:
- Is this an active or latent failure?
- Do you think the nurse is responsible?
- Can you identify the latent failures?

Using the '**5 WHY**' questions given, reflect on your practice experience and suggest possible explanations.

Consider the root cause of this error.

What can you learn from this?

When things have gone wrong for patients, one of the most valuable sources of information is the reports and voices of patients and carers (Berwick, 2013). One method of facilitating this is through patient stories. A patient story is an individual's description of their lived experience of their journey (or part of their journey) within healthcare delivery. Patient stories are acknowledged as a valuable and rich source of evidence within healthcare and healthcare education (Haigh and Hardy, 2011). They can be very powerful and memorable to those listening to them, as they offer insights into the patient journey that is implicit within the story. This can change listeners' understanding as the story resonates with their own experience and knowledge of the situation (Haigh and Hardy, 2011).

Patient stories can be positive, negative, or a combination of both. Opportunities to share learning through patient stories promotes active learning through reflective practice, rather than the transmission of knowledge. Reflective practice is integral to continuous learning and several evaluative reports support the concept of reflection when using patient stories (Christianson, 2011; Gidman, 2013). Christiansen (2011) also concluded that patient stories effectively promoted deep and critical engagement in student nurses. Together, they facilitated reflection, which improved their ability to gain new personal insights and self-appraisal of their own values, and beliefs about practice. It is beyond the remit of this chapter to explore reflection and reflective practice and you are encouraged to further your reading to understand the concepts of reflection and how it promotes continuous learning.

Patient stories can be captured through a variety of methods including patient feedback, written narratives and digital stories. Local NHS Trusts may use patient stories and it is worth exploring this in your clinical placements. There are also national websites that provide a range of digital patient stories (see below). You can review these individually and reflect upon your practice placement experiences. Alternatively, you may wish to share with your peers, tutors, your practice supervisor/assessor or with other members of the multidisciplinary teams.

Patient Voices: www.patientvoices.org.uk

Patient Stories: www.patientstories.org.uk

Patient Voices – Point of Care Foundation National Voices: www.pointofcare foundation.org.uk/resource/using-patient-experience-for-improvement/improving-care/patient-voices/

Activity 8.4 and the case study that follows use a digital patient story that relate to a patient safety incident. Both stories are very powerful and emotive to watch as they describe a catalogue of events as experienced by the patient and their family.

ACTIVITY 8.4

Methods of sharing patient stories can be one-to-one clinical supervision meetings, team meetings, group discussions, etc.

Take a look at the following patient story and share with other healthcare professionals.

Jimmy is a young man admitted to a mental health unit for treatment for depression. Jimmy has an unobserved fall that leads to a catalogue of events, resulting in a tragic ending for Jimmy and his relatives. His full story is told by his sister and available at www.patientvoices.org.uk/flv/0047pv384.htm

As a group consider the 5 WHYs:

Does this story resonate with current practice?

What are the positive and negative key themes in this story?

Identify any shared learning points and how these can be communicated widely so others can learn.

CASE STUDY: PATIENT SAFETY INCIDENT

Sepsis – a patient story (as told by Jeremy and his wife)

Jeremy was a self-employed 59-year-old man who had been diagnosed with a urinary tract infection (UTI) by his GP. He was treated with antibiotics, but his condition got progressively worse and Jeremy collapsed at home. He was rushed to the local A&E via ambulance with a severe UTI. On arrival, his symptoms were severe loin pain, pain on micturition and shortness of breath. In A&E he was seen by the doctor and spent 6 hours there before being transferred to a ward. During that time, his condition remained stable. Jeremy's wife (who we will name Ann) was very complimentary about the care delivered in the A&E Department.

On admission to the ward, Jeremy was reviewed by a doctor the following day and required continuous monitoring of his vital signs. Initially, he did not show any signs of deterioration, but 2 hours later Jeremy began to deteriorate. He had a respiratory rate of 32 rpm, a pulse rate of 132 beats per minute, blood pressure of 102/58 mmHg, and a temperature of 39°C. His National Early Warning Score (NEWS2) was 8 and he was deteriorating rapidly.

What would these vital signs indicate? What guidelines are in place when NEWS are escalating? What would you do in this situation?

Ann arrived at the hospital and noticed his deterioration, and Jeremy asked Ann if he should be on intravenous fluids and antibiotics. Ann went to see the nurse who told her that he should be on IV medication and fluids. Half an hour later, Jeremy had not commenced this treatment. Following continual persistence by Ann, Jeremy's treatment commenced. During his treatment, Jeremy's condition continued to deteriorate, pain increased (pain score of 9/10) and he felt nauseous. Ann voiced her concerns to three nurses and found that one nurse in particular reassured her that 'Jeremy was fine' and that 'She knew what she was doing'.

CASE STUDY: PATIENT SAFETY INCIDENT (*continued*)

There are a number of factors here relating to safety culture: what do you think they are?

Considering the responses by the nurse, what are the associated human factor elements causing delays in treatment?

Jeremy was eventually given repeated doses of morphine for his pain, which seemed to have the desired effect. However, Ann, knowing her husband well, became increasingly concerned as he began to go very quiet and calm. Ann felt that Jeremy was dying and voiced her concerns to the nurses but again, the nurse informed her that Jeremy was 'fine and they knew what they were doing' but nothing happened.

What is happening here? Do you know whether his vital signs have continued to be recorded? Do we know if his EWS has risen? Has this been escalated? How often do we listen to the voices of relatives? This is an important factor as she is telling the nurses that something is very wrong with Jeremy.

Eight hours later, after Jeremy had begun to dangerously deteriorate, a worried nurse called the hospital 'outreach team' for direct support. The outreach nurse arrived on the ward, took one look at Jeremy and immediately recognised that he was critically ill and needed urgent attention. Ann continued to repeatedly inform the outreach nurse that it was unusual for Jeremy to be ill. Jeremy was admitted to the Intensive Care Unit, sedated and commenced on IV antibiotics, high flow oxygen and medication to control his blood pressure.

Jeremy survived his illness and was later admitted to the ward, where he spent 5 months as an inpatient. He was later discharged home, but his illness resulted in life-changing circumstances.

This is clearly a patient safety incident resulting in severe harm to Jeremy and Ann.

Linking this to human factors, what active and latent failures would you consider to be the root cause? Is there a root cause? Or is this an active failure only?

What lessons can you learn from this incident? How will you disseminate and share this story with others?

The full story can be viewed on www.youtube.com/watch?v=Ch-XuVY_T9M

Summary

Nurses constitute the largest workforce in healthcare. They spend most time with patients and therefore play a vital role in patient safety. To improve patient safety, a positive safety culture must exist to protect patients from unnecessary harm. Safety culture is a multifaceted concept that incorporates many dimensions, but the fundamental element is communication, which has been discussed in this chapter. Understanding how harm does occur to patients, and reporting of errors so that lessons can be learnt, are vital to improving patient safety. A number of strategies and tools can be used to encourage learning from errors and more than one approach can be used. This chapter has focused on the use of patient stories as a method of learning from 'real life' clinical incidents and it is hoped that you can adopt this method to share with colleagues, peers and the wider healthcare teams.

Four key points to take away from *Chapter 8*:

- Effective communication in healthcare delivery is key to promoting patient safety and keeping patients from harm.
- The number of patient safety incidents continues to rise, and this could be contributory to a positive safety culture as today's healthcare systems and healthcare delivery foster the importance of incident reporting and applying a human factors approach to incidents.
- An open, transparent, human factors approach to patient safety incidents promotes a 'blame-free culture', which encourages reporting and learning from patient safety incidents.
- Reporting of incidents encourages learning from errors. A range of strategies can be employed and communicated within and across teams and the organisation. It is the responsibility of all healthcare professions to use and implement these strategies as this is critical to promoting a safer healthcare delivery and protecting patients from harm.

FURTHER READING

Bulman, C. and Schutz, S. (2016) *Reflective Practice in Nursing*, 5th edition. Wiley-Blackwell.

NHS England (2015) *Commissioning for Quality and Innovation (CQUIN): Guidance for 2015/16*. NHS England. Available at: www.england.nhs.uk/wp-content/uploads/2015/03/9-cquin-guid-2015-16.pdf (accessed 19 July 2019).

NHS Improvement (2013) *Safety Thermometer*. Available at: www.safety thermometer.nhs.uk

NHS Improvement (2018) *Learning from Patient Safety Incidents*. Available at: https://improvement.nhs.uk/resources/learning-from-patient-safety-incidents (accessed 19 July 2019).

REFERENCES

Agency for Healthcare Research and Quality (2012) *Hospital Survey on Patient Safety Culture: user's guide*. Available at: www.ahrq.gov/sites/default/files/wysiwyg/professionals/quality-patient-safety/patientsafetyculture/hospital/userguide/hospcult.pdf (accessed 19 July 2019).

Alahmadi, H.A. (2010) Assessment of patient safety culture in Saudi Arabian hospitals. *BMJ Quality and Safety*, **19(5)**: e17.

Berwick, D. (2013) *A Promise to Learn – A Commitment to Act: improving the safety of patients in England*. National Advisory Group on the Safety of Patients in England. Available at: https://assets.publishing.service.gov.uk/government/uploads/system/uploads/attachment_data/file/226703/Berwick_Report.pdf (accessed 19 July 2019).

Brasaite, I., Kaunonen, M. and Suominen, T. (2015) Healthcare professionals' knowledge, attitudes and skills regarding patient safety: a systematic literature review. *Scandinavian Journal of Caring Sciences*, **29**: 30–50.

Christiansen, A. (2011) Storytelling and professional learning: a phenomenographic study of students' experience of patient digital stories in nurse education. *Nurse Education Today*, **31**: 289–93.

Curry, L. and Nunez-Smith, M. (2015) *Mixed Methods in Health Sciences Research: a practical primer*. Sage Publications.

Department of Health (2000) *An Organisation with a Memory*. Stationery Office.

El-Jardali, F., Sheikh, F., Garcia, N.A., Jamal, D. and Abdo, A. (2014) Patient safety culture in a large teaching hospital in Riyadh: baseline assessment, comparative analysis and opportunities for improvement. *BMC Health Services Research*, **14(1)**: 1–15.

Gidman, J. (2013) Listening to stories: valuing knowledge from patient experience. *Nurse Education in Practice*, **13**: 192–6.

Haigh, C. and Hardy, P. (2011) Tell me a story – a conceptual exploration of storytelling in healthcare education. *Nurse Education Today*, **31**: 408–11.

Health and Safety Commission (1993) Third Report: Organising for Safety [cited in The Health Foundation (2013) *The Measurement and Monitoring of Safety*. Available at: www.health.org.uk/sites/default/ files/TheMeasurementAndMonitoringOfSafety_fullversion.pdf (accessed 19 July 2019).

Health and Safety Executive (1999) *Reducing Error and Influencing Behaviour*. HSE Books. Available at: www.hse.gov.uk/pUbns/priced/hsg48.pdf (accessed 19 July 2019).

Health Foundation (2013) *The Measurement and Monitoring of Safety*. Available at: www.health.org.uk/sites/default/files/TheMeasurement AndMonitoringOfSafety_fullversion.pdf (accessed 19 July 2019).

Keogh, B. (2013) *Review into the Quality of Care and Treatment Provided by 14 Hospital Trusts in England: overview report*. NHS England. Available at: www. nhs.uk/nhsengland/bruce-keogh-review/documents/outcomes/keogh-review-final-report.pdf (accessed 19 July 2019).

Kohn, L.T., Corrigan, J.M. and Donaldson, M.S. (2000) *To Err is Human: building a safer health system*. National Academic Press.

NHS Improvement (2018) *National Patient Safety Incident Reports: 27 March 2019*. Available at: https://improvement.nhs.uk/resources/national-patient-safety-incident-reports-27-march-2019/ (accessed 19 July 2019)

Nursing and Midwifery Council (2018a) *The Code: professional standards of practice and behaviour for nurses, midwives and nursing associates*. NMC. Available at: www.nmc.org.uk/globalassets/sitedocuments/nmc-publications/ nmc-code.pdf (accessed 19 July 2019).

Nursing and Midwifery Council (2018b) *Future Nurse: standards of proficiency for registered nurses*. NMC. Available at: www.nmc.org.uk/globalassets/ sitedocuments/education-standards/future-nurse-proficiencies.pdf (accessed 19 July 2019).

Reason, J. (1997) *Managing the Risks of Organizational Accidents*. Ashgate.

Royal College of Nursing (2017) *Communication*. Available at www.rcn.org.uk/clinical-topics/patient-safety-and-human-factors/professional-resources/communication (accessed 19 July 2019).

Sexton, J.B., Helmreich, R.L., Neilands, T.B. *et al.* (2006) The Safety Attitudes Questionnaire: psychometric properties, benchmarking data, and emerging research. *BMC Health Service Research*, **6(44)**: 1–10.

Taylor, J.B. (2012) *Safety Culture: assessing and changing the behaviour of organisations*. Gower Publishing Ltd.

Wang, X., Lui, L., Xiang, J. *et al.* (2014) The relationship between patient safety culture and adverse events: a questionnaire survey. *International Journal of Nursing Studies*, **51**: 1114–22.

Wears, R.L. (2012) Rethinking healthcare as a safety-critical industry. *Work*, **41(Suppl 1)**: 4560–3.

World Health Organization (2008) *Patient Safety Workshop: learning from error.* Available at: www.who.int/patientsafety/activities/technical/vincristine_learning-from-error.pdf (accessed 19 July 2019).

World Health Organization (2009) *Conceptual Framework for the International Classification for Patient Safety, Version 1.1: Final Technical Report (Technical Annex 2)*. Available at: www.who.int/patientsafety/taxonomy/icps_full_report.pdf (accessed 19 July 2019).

Index